EMS Field Guide®
ALS Version™

Nineteenth Edition

Meets the Most Current CPR and ECC Guidelines

- ★ 2010 AHA Updates
- ★ Medical Emergencies
- ★ Prescription Drugs
- ★ Spanish, Lab Values
- ★ Trauma, Triage, MCI
- ★ Updated ACLS Algorithms
- ★ 12-Lead ECGs, Acute MI
- ★ Pediatric Resuscitation
- ★ Emergency Medications

Paul LeSage, EMT-P, Assistant Chief
Paula Derr, RN, BSN, CCRN, CEN
Jon Tardiff, Paramedic, BS, PA-C

World Headquarters
Jones & Bartlett Learning
5 Wall Street
Burlington, MA 01803
978-443-5000
info@jblearning.com
www.jblearning.com

Jones & Bartlett Learning books and products are available through most bookstores and online booksellers. To contact Jones & Bartlett Learning directly, call 800-832-0034, fax 978-443-8000, or visit our website, www.jblearning.com.

Substantial discounts on bulk quantities of Jones & Bartlett Learning publications are available to corporations, professional associations, and other qualified organizations. For details and specific discount information, contact the special sales department at Jones & Bartlett Learning via the above contact information or send an email to specialsales@jblearning.com.

Copyright © 2011 by Jones & Bartlett Learning, LLC, an Ascend Learning Company

The procedures and protocols in this book are based on the most current recommendations of responsible medical sources. The publisher, however, makes no guarantee as to, and assumes no responsibility for, the correctness, sufficiency, or completeness of such information or recommendations. Other or additional safety measures may be required under particular circumstances.

This resource is intended solely as a guide to the appropriate procedures to be employed when rendering emergency care to the sick and injured. It is not intended as a statement of the standards of care required in any particular situation, because circumstances and the patient's physical condition can vary widely from one emergency to another. Nor is it intended that this resource shall in any way advise emergency personnel concerning legal authority to perform the activities or procedures discussed. Such local determination should be made only with the aid of legal counsel.

ISBN: 978-1-890495-57-2

6048

Printed in the United States of America
17 16 15   10 9 8 7 6 5 4

Radio/Phone Consultation

Identify: Unit #	Your Name
Patient Age	Sex
Chief Complaint (onset, duration, etc.)	
LOC	Level of Distress
Signs and Symptoms	
Pulse	BP
Respirations	Other
Skin	Pupils
Lung Sounds	ECG
Past Medical HX	
Medications	
Allergies	
Emergency Care	
Physician	
ETA	En Route Code
Time	Other

Airway

Rapid Sequence Intubation

Prepare equipment (IV, ECG, oximeter, BVM, suction, ETT); CO_2 detector; backup airway

↓

C-Spine immobilization, as needed

↓

Preoxygenate with 100% O_2; apply and maintain cricoid pressure

Place patient in sniff position; hyperventilate with O_2

↓

Give sedative
- Midazolam 0.1–0.3 mg/kg IV/IO OR:
- Thiopental 1–3 mg/kg IV/IO OR:
- Ketamine 1–2 mg/kg IV/IO OR:
- Etomidate 0.3 mg/kg IV/IO OR:
- Diazepam 0.2 mg/kg IV/IO (maximum 20 mg)

Lift tongue leftward and visualize vocal cords

↓

If patient <2 years old, **give Atropine 0.02 mg/kg IV/IO** (blocks reflex bradycardia)

↓

Give Succinylcholine 1–1.5 mg/kg IV/IO OR: Rocuronium 0.6–1.2 mg/kg IV/IO OR: Vecuronium 0.1 mg/kg IV/IO

Vocal cords

↓

Intubate (apply cricoid pressure, as needed)

↓

Inflate cuff; verify tube placement
- **Check chest expansion**
- **Check lung sounds**
- **Fogging of tube**
- **Apply CO_2 detector**
- **Secure with ETT holder and C-collar**

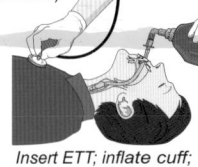

Insert ETT; inflate cuff; check breath sounds

King LT Airway

Contra—Patients <4 feet tall. Does not protect against aspiration.

1. **C-Spine immobilization**, as needed. **Preoxygenate with 100% O$_2$.** Apply water-based lube to distal tip and posterior aspect of tube.
2. **Deflate cuff. Open mouth, apply chin lift**, insert tip into side of mouth.
3. **Advance tip** behind tongue while rotating tube to midline.
4. **Advance tube** until base of connector is aligned with teeth or gums.
5. **Inflate cuff** with air (use minimum volume necessary).

Patient Size	LT Size	Cuff Vol
35–45 inches	Size 2	25–35 mL
41–51 inches	Size 2.5	30–40 mL
4–5 feet	Size 3	45–60 mL
5–6 feet	Size 4	60–80 mL
>6 feet	Size 5	70–90 mL

6. **Attach bag-valve device.** While ventilating, gently withdraw tube until ventilation becomes easy.
7. **Adjust cuff inflation**, if necessary, to obtain a good seal.
8. **Verify proper placement**
   - Check chest expansion and lung sounds
   - Apply CO_2 detector; oximeter
   - Secure with tape or tube holder
   - Reassess airway periodically

4

Trauma Triage Criteria

(For patient entry into the Trauma System.)

Physiological

- Systolic BP less than 90 mm/Hg
- Respiratory distress—rate <10 or >29
- Altered mental status, or Glasgow Coma Score ≤12

Anatomical

- Flail chest
- Two or more proximal long bone fractures (humerus, femur)
- Penetrating injuries to the head, neck, torso or groin; extremities proximal to elbow or knee
- Partial or full thickness burns to the face or airway
- Amputation proximal to the wrist or ankle
- Paralysis of any limb associated with trauma injury
- Pelvic fracture; open or depressed skull fracture; crushed, degloved, or mangled extremity

Mechanism

- Death of any occupant in the patient's vehicle
- Ejection of patient from an enclosed vehicle
- Falls greater than 20 feet (adult/10 feet; child/2–3 times child's height)
- Intrusion >12" occupant side or 18" any side
- Motorcycle crash >20 mph
- Auto/pedestrian or bicyclist thrown, run over, or with >20 mph impact
- Vehicle telemetry data consistent with high risk of injury

Comorbid Factors

Any combination of high-energy transfer in comorbid factor should increase the index of suspicion for severe trauma injury.
- Age <12 or >60
- Pregnancy
- Significant pre-existing medical problems

- Anticoagulation/bleeding disorder
- Burns with trauma
- Time-sensitive extremity injury
- End-stage renal disease needing dialysis
- EMS provider judgement

INDEX OF SUSPICION: You may enter any patient into the Trauma System suspected of having experienced significant trauma regardless of physical findings. Any combination of comorbid factors and high energy transfer is dangerous. The reason for system entry must be fully documented.

Notes

Rapid Triage

(For multiple patient scenes.)

Priority	Color	Condition	Notes
1	Red	Immediate	Life threatening
2	Yellow	Urgent	Can delay up to 1 hour
3	Green	Delayed	Up to 3 hours
4	Black	Deceased	No care needed

Priority 1—Immediate Transport

Unconscious, disoriented, very confused, rapid respirations, weak irregular pulse, severe uncontrolled bleeding, other signs of shock (cold, clammy skin, low blood pressure, etc.).

Priority 2—Urgent, Can Delay Transport Up To 1 hour

Conscious, oriented, with any significant fracture or other significant injury, but without signs of shock.

Priority 3—Delayed Transport Up To 3 hours

Walking wounded, CAO x3, minor injuries.

Priority 4—Deceased, No Care Needed

No pulse, no respirations (open airway first), obvious mortal wounds (e.g., decapitation).

NOTE: Assessment of patients should be <15 seconds each. (Have someone else control bleeding during your survey.)
• All unconscious patients are **Priority 1**—Immediate
• "Walking wounded" are usually **GREEN**—Priority 3
• All pulseless patients are **BLACK**—Priority 4

Mentation/LOC Assessment

A—Alert	Able to answer questions.
V—Verbal	Responds to verbal stimuli.
P—Pain	Responds only to pain stimuli. Protect airway.
U—Unconscious	Protect airway, consider intubation.

Multiple Patients

1. Strategically park vehicle and stay in one place

2. **Establish Command**, and identify yourself as Command to dispatch (use a calm, clear voice)

3. **Size up the scene** and advise dispatch of:
   - Exact location and type of incident
   - Estimated number and severity of patients
   - Any hazardous conditions
   - The best routes of access to the scene
   - The location of the command post

4. **Designate an EMT to perform rapid triage** (see *Trauma section, Rapid Triage*, for more contraindications), tag and number multiple patients ("Immediate," "Urgent," "Delayed")

5. **Order resources** (Fire, Police, Ambulances, HazMat, Extrication, Air Units, Tow vehicles, Buses, etc.)

6. **Set up staging areas** (clearly state the location of staging/assembly areas, and think of access and egress)

7. **Coordinate access** of incoming units to the scene

8. **Assign patients** to incoming medical units

9. **Maintain communications** with On-Line Medical Control (OLMC)

10. **Keep patient log** indicating patient number, name, severity, treating and transporting units, medical interventions, and destination hospitals

Mass Casualty Incident

NOTE: Use Multiple Patient guidelines above, and the following ICS groups.

Medical Branch Director

- Reports to IC
- Responsible for overall medical direction/coordination
- Orders additional medical resources
- Serves as a resource for group supervisors

Triage Group Supervisor

- Estimates number and severity of patients
- Establishes tagging and extrication teams
- Establishes triage areas, if necessary
- Maintains rapid and orderly flow of patients to treatment areas

Treatment Area Group Supervisor

- Secures treatment areas, identifies equipment needs
- Clearly marks Treatment Areas for "Immediate," "Urgent," "Delayed"
- Establishes treatment teams when resources allow
- Identifies order of patient transport

Transportation Group Supervisor

- Establishes Patient Loading Zone (near Treatment Area)
- Assigns patients to ambulances, supervises actual loading
- Relays Unit number, severity and number of patients to Communications Group Supervisor

Communications Group Supervisor

- Communicates with On-line Medical Control (OLMC) to identify receiving hospitals
- Maintains patient log
- Receives information from Transportation Group
- Coordinates patient destinations to avoid overloading the closest hospitals

Abbreviations Used In This Section

HX—History, Signs, and Symptoms
Key Symptoms and Findings (green text)
➕—Prehospital Treatment (blue text with yellow background)
Cautions—Contraindications or Precautions (red text)

Trauma—Abdominal

HX—Mechanism of injury, associated trauma, penetrating vs. blunt injury? Suspect internal hemorrhage. **Guarding, distension, rigidity, hypotension, pallor, bruising?**
➕—Vitals, O_2, IV, treat for shock, transport.

Trauma—Burns

HX—Airway burns (soot in mouth, red mouth, singed nasal hairs, **cough, hoarseness, dyspnea**)? Was patient in enclosed space? How long? **Did patient lose consciousness?** Was there an explosion? Toxic fumes? Hx cardiac or lung disease? Estimate % of burns and depth. Other trauma?

NOTE: Significant burns = blistered or charred areas, or burns of the hands, feet, face, airway, genitalia.

➕—**Stop the burning**: Extinguish clothing if smouldering.
- Remove clothing, if not adhered to skin; remove jewelry.
- Vitals, give high flow O_2, assist ventilations if needed.
- ❖ **Superficial and Deep Superficial Burns**: If <20%, apply wet dressings.
- ❖ **Moderate to Severe Burns**: Cover with dry sterile dressing (DSD) and/or burn sheet. Leave blisters intact. Start large bore IV, treat for shock or % burn. Monitor ECG.
- ❖ **Chemical Burns**: Brush off any dry chemical then flush with copious amounts of water or saline.
  For lime: Brush off excess, then flush; For phosphorus: Use **copious** amounts of water.
- ❖ **Electrical Burns**: Apply DSD to entry and exit wounds. Start large bore IV, titrate for shock. Monitor ECG—treat dysrhythmias per ACLS.

Cautions—Consider child abuse in pediatric patients.

10

Trauma

WARNING: Do not apply ointments to burns. Avoid starting IV in burned area if possible. Consider carbon monoxide (CO) poisoning. Pulse oximetry not accurate with CO.

IMPORTANT: Burned firefighters may be having an AMI.

Burn Chart

NOTE: Count only second degree and third degree burns.

Infant

18

10

16 Front
16 Rear

10

14   1   14

Adult

9

18 Front
18 Rear

9   9

1

18   18

IV FLUID RESUSCITATION*

$$\frac{\% \text{ Burn Area} \times \text{Pt. Wt. in Kg}}{4} = \text{mL/hour NS}$$

Give this amount over the first 8 hours;
Give an equal amount over the next 16 hours.

Example: 20% burned area, patient weighs 70 kg:

$$\frac{20 \times 70}{4} = \frac{1400}{4} = 350 \text{ mL/hour for 8 hours}^\dagger$$

Then give 175 mL/hour over the next 16 hours. †(calculated from time of injury)

*The patient in shock needs more aggressive IV fluid replacement and should be treated according to your shock protocol.

NOTE: Major burns should be treated in a burn center, including: ≥25% body surface; hands, feet, face, or perineum; electrical burns; inhalation burns; other injuries; or severe pre-existing medical problems.

Trauma—Cardiac Arrest
(See ACLS section, Trauma Cardiac Arrest algorithm)

NOTE: Rapid extrication and transport immediately.

✚—Secure airway, do CPR (shock VF), O_2, IVs en route. Splint fractures en route.

Trauma—Chest

NOTE: Suspect cardiac, pulmonary, or great vessel trauma.

✚—Secure airway, high flow O_2, intubate if necessary and assist ventilations. **Open chest wound**: cover with occlusive dressing. Look for exit wounds. **Tension pneumothorax**: evaluate and decompress. **Impaled objects**: stabilize in place. Do not delay transport if patient is unstable. Consider IV fluids for shock (2 large bore IVs), monitor ECG, vitals. Full spinal immobilization.

Cautions—Consider other causes for respiratory distress.

Notes

Trauma—Crush Injury with Entrapment

NOTE: While crushed, the patient's BP, HR, and RR may appear normal. Sudden release can cause reperfusion syndrome (Crush Syndrome).

⊞—Give patient dust mask or O_2 mask (humidified best), treat for hypothermia, start IV fluids BEFORE crush mechanism lifted, especially if crushed >4 hours. If IV fluids not possible, consider short-term use of tourniquet on affected limb until IV hydration initiated. Safety glasses and noise protection, as needed.

PREVENT:
- **Hypotension**: a result of third spacing and hemorrhage
- **Renal failure**: IV fluids, mannitol, dialysis
- **Acidosis**: sodium bicarbonate
- **Hyperkalemia/hypocalcemia**: consider calcium, insulin, D50 and kayexalate with sorbitol
- **Cardiac arrhythmia**: treat accordingly to ACLC guidelines; monitor for pain, pallor, parasthesias, pain with passive movement, pulselessness

CAUTION: If >1 hour of crush, do not release crushing mechanism until ready.

Trauma—Head

⊞—Secure airway while providing C-spine immobilization. Control bleeding with direct pressure. Do not stop bleeding from nose, ears if CSF leak is suspected, O_2, IV (TKO unless patient is in shock). Monitor vitals and neuro status. ECG, oximetry; consider intubation and ventilation if GCS ≤8. Hyperventilate to ETCO$_2$ of 30–35. Elevate HOB 15°–30°.

Cautions—Always suspect C-spine injury in the head injury patient. Assess and document LOC changes. Be alert for airway problems and seizures. Restlessness and or agitation can be due to hypoxia or hypoglycemia. Check Chemstrip®.

Glasgow Coma Scale

NOTE: Patient with a score of 3–8 is in a coma and needs ventilatory support.

Eye Opening

INFANT			CHILD/ADULT
4	Spontaneously	Spontaneously	4
3	To speech	To command	3
2	To pain	To pain	2
1	No response	No response	1

Best Verbal Response

5	Coos, babbles	Oriented	5
4	Irritable cries	Confused	4
3	Cries to pain	Inappropriate words	3
2	Moans, grunts	Incomprehensible	2
1	No response	No response	1

Best Motor Response

6	Spontaneous	Obeys commands	6
5	Localizes pain	Localizes pain	5
4	Withdraws from pain	Withdraws from pain	4
3	Flexion (decorticate)	Flexion (decorticate)	3
2	Extension (decerebrate)	Extension (decereb.)	2
1	No response	No response	1

___ = Total →(GCS ≤8? →Intubate!) ← Total = ___

Trauma

Trauma—Spinal Injury

HX—MOI, helmet worn? Suspect C-spine injury with head or neck trauma, and with multi-system trauma, or diving/drowning. Altered mental status? Is there paralysis, weakness, numbness, tingling? Spinal pain with or without movement, point tenderness, deformity, or guarding?

✚—Keep airway open. Consider nasopharyngeal airway. Splint neck with C-collar and immobilize the entire spine. Move the patient as a unit and only as necessary. Give O_2, Start large bore IV. Vitals. **Place patient in Trauma System**.

Cautions—Be prepared to suction and/or move the patient as a unit while immobilized. Consider internal bleeding.

Spinal Innervation

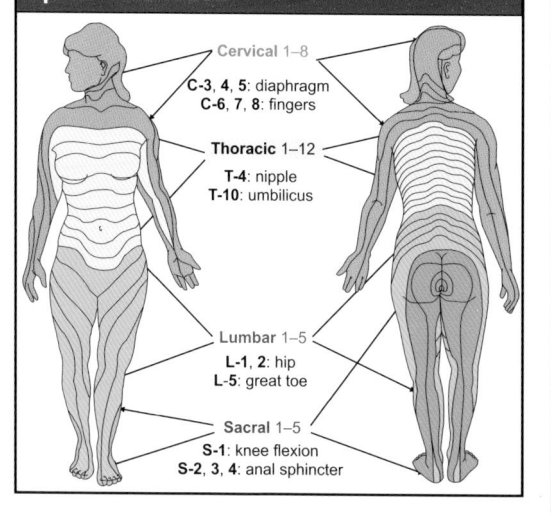

Cervical 1–8
C-3, 4, 5: diaphragm
C-6, 7, 8: fingers

Thoracic 1–12
T-4: nipple
T-10: umbilicus

Lumbar 1–5
L-1, 2: hip
L-5: great toe

Sacral 1–5
S-1: knee flexion
S-2, 3, 4: anal sphincter

ACLS Algorithms

NOTE: ECGs illustrated in this guide are for reference only and should not be interpreted as exact.

NOTE: Not all patients require the treatment indicated by these algorithms. These algorithms assume that you have assessed the patient, started CPR where indicated, and performed reassessment after each treatment. These algorithms also do not exclude other appropriate interventions which may be warranted by the patient's condition. **Treat the patient, not the ECG.**

Notes

Cardiac Arrest

Shout for help, begin CPR (30:2, push hard and fast at ≥100/minute, minimize interruptions), **give O₂, attach ECG.**

YES ⇦ Shockable Rhythm? ⇨ NO

VF or VT	Asystole/PEA

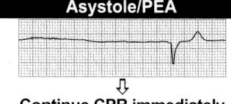

VF or VT

⇩

〜**Defibrillate 120 J–200 J Biphasic** (or 360 J monophasic, or AED)

⇩

Continue CPR immediately x2 minutes. Start IV/IO.

⇩

VF/VT?

⇩

〜**Defibrillate**
Continue CPR x2 minutes.
Epinephrine 1 mg IV/IO, repeat every 3–5 minutes, *OR:*
Vasopressin 40 Units IV/IO (single dose only)
Consider advanced airway (ET Tube, supraglottic airway)
Ventilate 8–10 breaths/minute with continuous compressions.
Use waveform capnography: If PETCO₂ <15, improve CPR.

⇩

VF/VT?

⇩

〜**Defibrillate**
Continue CPR x2 minutes.
Amiodarone 300 mg IV/IO, (may repeat once 150 mg in 5 minutes)
Consider Reversible Causes. ❖

⇩

If ROSC (pulse, BP, PETCO₂ ≥40 mm Hg), see *ROSC algorithm,* next page.

Asystole/PEA

⇩

Continue CPR immediately x2 minutes. Start IV/IO.
Epinephrine 1 mg IV/IO, repeat every 3–5 minutes, *OR:*
Vasopressin 40 Units IV/IO (single dose only) **Consider advanced airway** (ET Tube, supraglottic airway)
Ventilate 8–10 breaths/min. with continuous compressions.
Use waveform capnography: If PETCO₂ <15, improve CPR.

⇩

Asystole/PEA?

⇩

Continue CPR x2 minutes.
Consider Reversible Causes. ❖

⇩

If ROSC (pulse, BP, PETCO₂ ≥40 mm Hg), see *ROSC algorithm,* next page.

❖**Reversible Causes:**
- Hypoxia
- Hypovolemia
- Acidosis
- Hyper/Hypokalemia
- Hypothermia
- Coronary Thrombosis
- Cardiac Tamponade
- Tension Pneumothorax
- Toxins

Return of Spontaneous Circulation: Post Cardiac Arrest Care

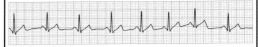

Optimize Ventilation/Oxygenation
(start at 10–12 breaths per minute, but *do not hyperventilate*)
Goal: PETCO$_2$ 35–40 mm Hg.
Use minimum amount of FiO$_2$ to keep SaO$_2$ ≥94%
Consider waveform capnography
⇩

Keep blood pressure ≥90 mm Hg (or MAP ≥65)
IV fluid bolus: 1–2 Liter(s) NS or RL
(may use cold [4°C] IV fluid if induced hypothermia)

> **Consider vasopressor infusion**
> **Epinephrine: 0.1–0.5 mcg/kg/minute**
> **Dopamine: 5–10 mcg/kg/minute**
> **Norepinephrine: 0.1–0.5 mcg/kg/minute**

Consider Reversible Causes❖
Monitor ECG, obtain 12-lead ECG
⇩
Follows commands?
(if not, consider induced hypothermia)
⇩
STEMI or High suspicion AMI?
⇩
Coronary reperfusion (PCI)
Advanced critical care

❖Reversible Causes:

- Hypoxia
- Acidosis
- Hypovolemia
- Toxins
- Coronary Thrombosis

- Cardiac Tamponade
- Hyper/Hypokalemia
- Hypothermia
- Pulmonary Thrombosis
- Tension Pneumothorax

Bradycardia
(HR <50/minute with serious S/Sx: shock, hypotension, altered
mental status, ischemic chest pain, acute heart failure.)

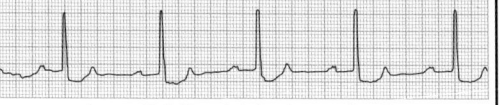

Assess C-A-B, **maintain airway, give O$_2$,**
assist breathing if needed. Attach pulse oximeter, BP cuff,
12-lead ECG, start IV/IO.
Consider and Treat Reversible Causes❖
⇩
Atropine 0.5 mg IV/IO every 3–5 minutes, maximum: 3 mg
(Do not delay TCP while starting IV, or waiting for
Atropine to work*.) *If ineffective:*
⇩
Transcutaneous Pacing (verify capture and perfusion;
use sedation as needed) *OR:*
Dopamine 2–10 mcg/kg per minute, *OR:*
Epinephrine 2–10 mcg per minute
⇩
Consider expert consult; prepare for transvenous pacer
⇩
Cardiac Arrest? —See *ACLS section, Cardiac Arrest Algorithm*
⇩

❖**Reversible Causes**:	*Atropine may not work for
• Hypoxia	transplanted hearts, Mobitz
• Acidosis	(Type II) AV Block or third
• Hypovolemia	degree AV Block with IVR.
• Toxins	
• Coronary Thrombosis	
• Cardiac Tamponade	
• Hyper/Hypokalemia	
• Hypothermia	—Begin pacing, and/or
• Pulmonary Thrombosis	catecholamine infusion.
• Tension Pneumothorax	

UNSYMPTOMATIC BRADYCARDIA?
— NOT Type II (Mobitz) second degree or third degree
AV heart block?
⇩
Observe

Notes

Tachycardias

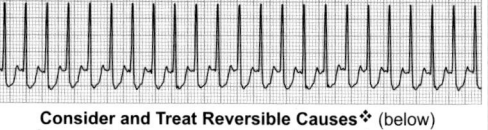

Consider and Treat Reversible Causes❖ (below)
Assess C-A-B, secure airway, give O$_2$, start IV/IO,
check BP, apply Oximeter, get 12-lead ECG

Is Patient Unstable?	Stable?

(Serious S/Sx must be related to the tachycardia: Go to next
HR ≥150, ischemic chest pain, dyspnea, ↓LOC, page
↓BP, shock, heart failure.)

↗Immediate Synchronized Cardioversion
(for narrow QRS, consider Adenosine 6 mg, rapid IVP
(flush with NS, may repeat with 12 mg IVP); **also
consider sedation**, but do not delay cardioversion)
Initial Energy Doses: (if unsuccessful, increase
doses in a stepwise fashion.)
Narrow QRS, Regular: 50 J–100 J
Narrow QRS, Irregular: 120 J–200 J biphasic,
(or 200 J monophasic)
Wide QRS, Regular: 100 J
Wide QRS, Irregular: defibrillate with 120 J–200 J
biphasic, (or 360 J monophasic)

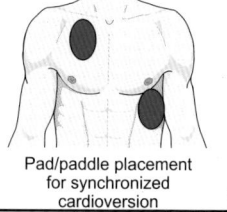

Synchronize Markers

Pad/paddle placement
for synchronized
cardioversion

Synchronize on R wave

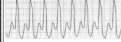

Stable Patient, Wide QRS (≥0.12 seconds)	Stable Patient, Narrow QRS
• 12-lead ECG • Start IV • **Consider Adenosine 6 mg IVP** (for regular, monomorphic rhythm) flush with saline, may repeat 12 mg IVP • **Consider antiarrhythmic:** *Either:* Procainamide 20–50 mg/minute IV until rhythm converts, QRS widens by 50%, hypotension, or maximum dose 17 mg/kg. Avoid if CHF or prolonged QT. Drip 1–4 mg/minute *OR:* Amiodarone 150 mg IV over 10 minutes. May repeat, (maximum dose: 2.2 gm IV/24 hours). Drip 1 mg/minute *OR:* Sotalol 1.5 mg/kg IV over 5 min. Avoid if prolonged QT. • **Consult with expert**	• 12-lead ECG • Start IV • **Vagal maneuvers*** • **Adenosine 6 mg IVP** (for regular rhythm) flush with saline, may repeat 12 mg IVP *Either:* • **Calcium blocker** (choose one:) Verapamil 2.5–5 mg IV over 2–3 minutes. May repeat 5–10 mg. Maximum 30 mg. Diltiazem 0.25 mg/kg IV over 2 minutes. May repeat 0.35 mg/kg. *OR:* • **Beta blocker** (choose one:) Metoprolol 5 mg IV over 2–5 minutes. May repeat. Maximum 15 mg. Atenolol 5 mg IV over 5 minutes. May repeat once. Propranolol 1–3 mg IV slowly over 2–5 minutes. Esmolol 250–500 mcg/kg x1 minute. • **Consult with expert**

❖**Reversible Causes:**
- Hypoxia
- Acidosis
- Hypovolemia
- Toxins
- Coronary Thrombosis
- Cardiac Tamponade
- Hyper/Hypokalemia
- Hypothermia
- Pulmonary Thrombosis
- Tension Pneumothorax

*Carotid sinus massage is contraindicated in patients with carotid bruits. Avoid ice application to face, if patient has ischemic heart disease.

Asthma Cardiac Arrest

Use standard ACLS Guidelines
Endotracheal intubation via RSI
(use largest ET tube possible; monitor waveform capnography)

⇩

To reduce hyperinflation, hypotension, and risk of tension pneumothorax, consider:
- Ventilate with a slower respiratory rate
- Smaller tidal volume (6–8 mL/kg)
- Shorter inspiratory time (80–100 mL/minute)
- Longer expiratory time (I/E 1:4 or 1:5)

⇩

Continue inhaled beta₂ agonist (albuterol)
via ET tube
Evaluate for tension pneumothorax

⇩

Consult with expert

⇩

Consider: brief disconnect from BVM and
press on chest wall during exhalation
to relieve air trapping

⇩

If the patient suddenly deteriorates

⇩

DOPE:
- **Displacement of ETT**
- **Obstruction of tube**
- **Pneumothorax**
- **Equipment failure**
- **Evaluate for Auto-PEEP**

Cardiac Arrest During PCI

- Consider mechanical CPR
- Consider emergency cardiopulmonary bypass
- Consider Cough CPR
- Consider intracoronary verapamil for reperfusion induced Ventricular Tachycardia

Cardiac Tamponade Cardiac Arrest

- Emergency pericardiocentesis
- Consider emergency department thoracotomy

Drowning Cardiac Arrest

- Begin rescue breathing ASAP
- **Start CPR with A-B-C** (Airway and Breathing first)
- **Anticipate vomiting** (have suction ready)
- **Attach AED** (dry chest off with towel)
- **Check for hypothermia**
- Use Standard BLS and ACLS

Electrocution Cardiac Arrest

(Respiratory arrest is common)

- Is the scene safe?
- Triage patients and treat those with respiratory arrest or cardiac arrest first
- **Start CPR**
- **Stabilize the cervical spine**
- **Attach AED**
- **Remove smoldering clothing**
- **Check for trauma**
- **Large bore IV for rapid fluid administration**
- **Consider early intubation for airway burns**
- Use Standard BLS and ACLS

Electrolyte Imbalance Cardiac Arrest

Hyperkalemia:

Wide QRS, peaked T waves, IVR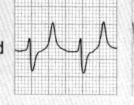

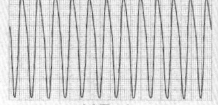

V-Tach

Calcium chloride 10% 500–1,000 mg IV/IO (5–10 mL) over 2–5 minutes [or calcium gluconate 10% 15–30 mL over 2–5 minutes].
Sodium bicarbonate 50 mEq IV/IO over 5 minutes [may repeat in 15 minutes]
Dextrose 25 grams (50 mL of D50) IV/IO + Regular Insulin 10 Units IV/IO over 15–30 minutes
Albuterol 10–20 mg nebulized over 15 minutes
Furosemide 40–80 mg IV/IO

Hypokalemia: Use Standard BLS and ACLS

Long QT interval, flat T waves, U wave

Hypermagnesemia:

Stop magnesium infusion
Consider: **Calcium chloride 10% 500–1,000 mg IV/IO** (5–10 mL) over 2–5 minutes [or calcium gluconate 10% 15–30 mL over 2–5 minutes]

Hypomagnesemia: Magnesium sulfate 1–2 grams IV/IO

Polymorphic VT (Torsades)

Pulmonary Embolism Cardiac Arrest

(Pulseless electrical activity is common)

- Standard BLS and ACLS
- **Emergency echocardiography**
- **Fibrinolytic for presumed PE**
- **Consult expert**
- **Consider percutaneous mechanical thrombectomy or surgical embolectomy**

Trauma Cardiac Arrest

Consider Reversible Causes❖ (below)

- Stabilize cervical spine
- **Jaw thrust to open airway**
- **Direct pressure for hemorrhage**
- Standard CPR and defibrillation
- **Use advanced airway if BVM inadequate** (consider cricothyrotomy if ventilation impossible)
- **Administer IV fluids** for hypovolemia
- Consider resuscitative thoracotomy

❖**Reversible Causes:**

• Hypoxia	• Cardiac Tamponade
• Acidosis	• Hyper/Hypokalemia
• Hypovolemia	• Hypothermia
• Toxins	• Pulmonary Thrombosis
• Coronary Thrombosis	• Tension Pneumothorax

"**Commotio Cordis**": a blow to the anterior chest causing VF
- Prompt CPR and defibrillation
- Standard BLS and ACLS

Hypothermia

- Remove wet clothing and stop heat loss (cover with blankets and insulating equipment)
- Keep patient horizontal
- Move patient gently, if possible; do not jostle
- Monitor core temperature and cardiac rhythm
- Treat underlying causes (drug overdose, alcohol, trauma, etc.) simultaneously with resuscitation
- Check responsiveness, breathing, pulse

If Pulse and Breathing	No Pulse/Apneic
34°C–36°C 93°F–97°F (MILD hypothermia) Passive rewarming	**Start CPR, Ventilate Defibrillate VF/VT Biphasic: 120 J–200 J OR: Monophasic 360 J Resume CPR Immediately** [Consider further defibrillation attempts for VF/VT] *See ACLS section, Cardiac Arrest algorithm.*
30°C–34°C 86°F–93°F (MODERATE hypothermia) Active external rewarming forced-air rewarming	Intubate, ventilate with warm, humid oxygen (42°C–46°C) Start IV/IO, administer warm normal saline (43°C) [Consider vasopressor: epinephrine 1 mg IV every 3–5 minutes, *OR:* vasopressin 40 Units IV]
<30°C <86°F (SEVERE hypothermia) Core rewarming (cardiopulmonary bypass, thoracic cavity warm water lavage, extracorporeal blood warming with partial bypass)	⇩ Continue CPR, Transport to ED, start core rewarming when feasible. Continue resuscitation until patient is rewarmed.
Adjunctive rewarming: • Warm IV fluids (43°C) • Warm, humid O$_2$ (42°C–46°C) • Peritoneal lavage • Extracorporeal rewarming • Esophageal rewarming tubes • Endovascular rewarming	⇩ After ROSC, rewarm patient to 32°C–34°C (90°F–93°F), or to normal body temperature.

Stemi Fibrinolytic Protocol
"Time is muscle"

"Door-to-Drug" time should be <30 minutes.

- **S/S:** Cx pain >15 minute, but <12 hours.
- **Get Stat 12-lead ECG.** (Must show ST elevation, or new LBBB.)
- ECG and other findings consistent with AMI.
- **Give:** O_2, **NTG**, Morphine, **ASA** (if no contraindications).
- **Start 2 IVs** (but do not delay transport).
- **Systolic/diastolic BP: Right arm ___/___ Left arm___/___.**
- **Complete Fibrinolytic Checklist** (all should be "No"):
  - ❏ Systolic BP >180–200 mm Hg
  - ❏ Diastolic BP >100–110 mm Hg
  - ❏ Right arm vs. left arm BP difference >15 mm Hg
  - ❏ Stroke >3 hours or <3 months
  - ❏ Hx Structural CNS Disease
  - ❏ Head/Facial Trauma within 3 weeks
  - ❏ Major trauma, GI/GU bleed, or surgery within 4 weeks
  - ❏ On blood thinners; bleeding/clotting problems
  - ❏ Pregnancy
  - ❏ History intracranial hemorrhage
  - ❏ Advanced cancer, severe liver/renal disease

High-Risk Profile/Indications for Transfer:

(if any are checked, consider transport to a hospital capable of angiography and revascularization)

- ❏ Heart rate ≥100 bpm and SBP ≤100 mm Hg
- ❏ Pulmonary edema (rales)
- ❏ Signs of shock
- ❏ Received CPR
- ❏ Contraindications to fibrinolytics

*If no contraindications and Dx of AMI is confirmed:

Administer fibrinolytic. Also consider: **anticoagulants**, and **standard ACS treatments.** *Signs of reperfusion include:* pain relief, ST-segment normalization, reperfusion dysrhythmias, resolution of conduction block, early cardiac marker peak.

3-Lead and MCL₁ Electrode Placement

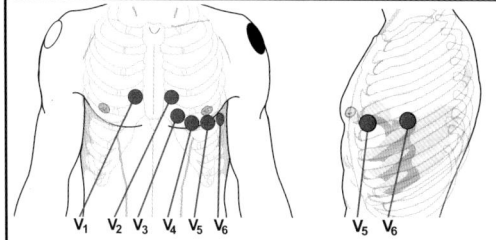

White Lead I Black

MCL₁

Lead III

Lead II

Red (on thigh↓)

-150° avR avL -30°

I 0°

III avF II

120° 90° 60°

12-Lead Electrode Placement

V₁ V₂ V₃ V₄ V₅ V₆   V₅ V₆

V₁: 4th interspace, just to the right of the sternum
V₂: 4th interspace, just to the left of the sternum
V₃: halfway between V₂ and V₄
V₄: 5th intercostal space, midclavicular line
V₅: anterior-axillary line, horizontal with V₄
V₆: mid-axillary line, horizontal with V₄
MCL₁: red lead on V₁, black lead on left arm—monitor lead III
MCL₆: red lead on V₆, white lead on right arm—monitor lead II
MC₄R: red lead on 5th ICS right mid-clavicular line, black lead on left arm—monitor lead III

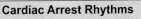

Cardiac Arrest Rhythms

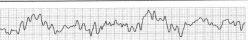

Coarse Ventricular Fibrillation
(Note the chaotic, irregular electrical activity) **Treatment**: Shock

Fine Ventricular Fibrillation
(Note the low-amplitude, irregular electrical activity)
Treatment: Shock

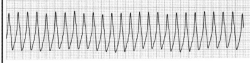

Ventricular Tachycardia
(Note the rapid, wide complexes) **Treatment**: Shock if no pulse

Asystole
(Note the absence of electrical activity) **Treatment**: Perform CPR

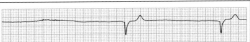

Pulseless Electrical Activity (PEA)
(Any organized ECG rhythm with no pulse)
Treatment: Perform CPR

ACLS

Other Common ECG Rhythms

Normal Sinus Rhythm
(Note the regular PQRST cycles)

fibrillatory
waves

Atrial Fibrillation
(Note the irregular rate and atrial fibrillatory waves)

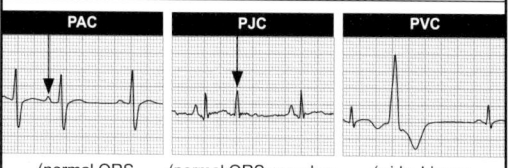

PAC	PJC	PVC
(normal QRS complex; different P wave)	(normal QRS complex; inverted or no P wave)	(wide, bizarre complex; no P wave)

Premature Atrial, Junctional, and Ventricular Complexes

Other Common ECG Rhythms

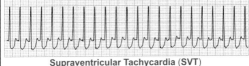

Supraventricular Tachycardia (SVT)
(Note the rapid, narrow QRS complexes)

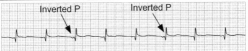

Inverted P   Inverted P

Junctional Rhythm
(Normal QRS complexes; inverted, or no P waves)

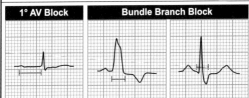

1° AV Block	Bundle Branch Block

(Prolonged PR Interval >0.20 seconds)   (Wide QRS >0.12 seconds)

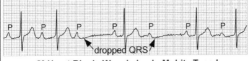

P   P   P   P   P   P   P

dropped QRS

2° Heart Block, Wenckebach, Mobitz Type I
(The PR interval lengthens, resulting in a dropped QRS)

Other Common ECG Rhythms

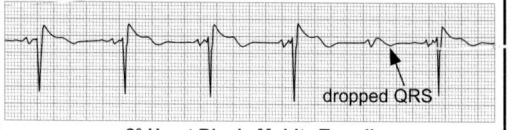

2° Heart Block, Mobitz Type II
(The PR interval does not lengthen; but a QRS is dropped)

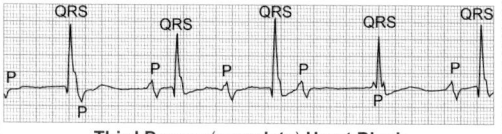

Third Degree (complete) Heart Block
(The P waves are dissociated from the QRS complexes)

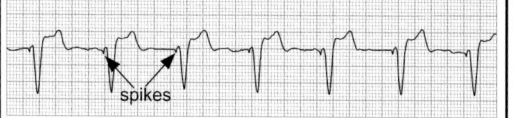

Electronic Ventricular Pacemaker
(Note the pacer spikes before each QRS)

Rapid Interpretation—12-Lead ECG

❶ Identify the rhythm. If supraventricular (Sinus Rhythm, Atrial Fibrillation, Atrial Tachycardia, Atrial Flutter):

❷ Rule out LBBB (QRS >0.12 seconds; and R–R' in I, or V_5, or V_6). LBBB confounds the Dx of AMI/ACS (unless it is new-onset LBBB).

LBBB

❸ If no LBBB, check for ST segment elevation, *OR* ST depression with T wave inversion, *OR* pathologic Q waves.

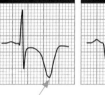

ST elevation	T wave inversion	Wide or deep QS

❹ Means acute MI · **May mean myocardial ischemia, or impending MI** · **Means infarction**

❺ Rule out other confounders: WPW (mimics infarct, BBB), pericarditis (mimics MI), digoxin (depresses STs), LVH (depresses STs, inverts T)

❻ Identify location of infarct and consider appropriate treatments (MONA, PCI [or fibrinolytic], nitrate infusion, heparin, GP IIb, IIIa inhibitor, beta blockers, antiarrhythmic, etc.)

ACLS

Normal 12-Lead ECG

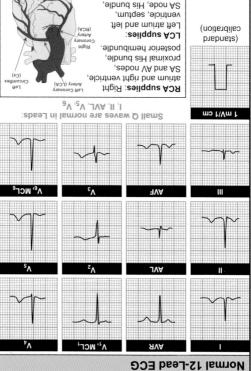

Small Q waves are normal in Leads:
I, II, AVL, V_5, V_6

RCA supplies: Right
atrium and right ventricle,
SA and AV nodes,
proximal His bundle,
posterior hemibundle.

LCA supplies:
Left ventricle, septum,
SA node, His bundle,
right and left bundle
branches, anterior and.
posterior hemibundles.

Right Anterior Descending (LAD)

Right Coronary Artery (RCA)

Left Circumflex (Cx)

Left Coronary Artery (LCA)

1 mV/1 cm

(standard calibration)

Myocardial Infarction ECG Patterns

(If signs of AMI are not present on the initial ECG perform serial ECGs.)

Injury	Ischemia	Acute Infarction
(ST segments usually elevate within minutes of the onset of cardiac chest pain)	(T waves invert fully by 24 hours)	(Pathologic Q waves ≥.03 seconds or 1/3 height of QRS begin to form in 1 hour)

Old Infarction		
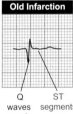		
Q waves remain forever ST segments are normal	**Reciprocal ST Depression** (found in leads away from the infarction)	**Non-Q-Wave Infarction** (flat, depressed ST segments in two or more contiguous leads; or may have inverted T waves)

NOTE: Early reperfusion is the definitive treatment for most AMI patients. The patient can lose 1% of salvageable myocardium for each minute of delay. Remember: "Time is Muscle."

Acute Anterior MI

(ST segment elevation ≥0.5–1 mm, with or without Q waves in two or more contiguous Leads: V_1–V_4. Poor R wave progression* and inverted T waves may also be present. Reciprocal ST depression may be present in: II, III, AVF.)

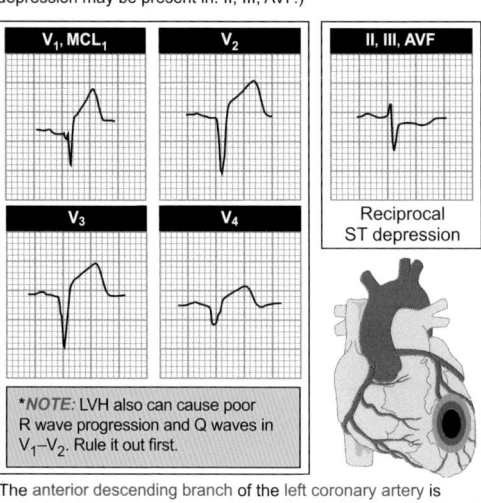

V_1, MCL_1	V_2	II, III, AVF

V_3	V_4	Reciprocal ST depression

*NOTE: LVH also can cause poor R wave progression and Q waves in V_1–V_2. Rule it out first.

The anterior descending branch of the left coronary artery is occluded. May cause: left anterior hemiblock; right bundle branch block; 2° AV block Mobitz II, 3° AV block with IVR, pump failure.

Third Degree Block

Acute Inferior MI

(ST segment elevation ≥0.5–1 mm in two or more contiguous Leads: II, III, AVF. Q waves and inverted T waves may also be present. Reciprocal ST depression may be present in Leads: I, AVL, V_2–V_4.)

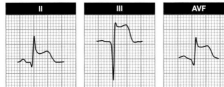

II	III	AVF

I, AVL	V_2, V_3, V_4

Reciprocal ST depression

NOTE: Right ventricle AMI accompanies Inferior AMI 30% of the time. Check lead V_4R for elevated ST segment and Q wave.

The right (or left) coronary artery is occluded. May cause: left posterior hemiblock; left axis deviation, ↓BP, sinus bradycardia, 1° AV block, 2° AV block Mobitz I (Wenckebach), 3° AV block with IJR.

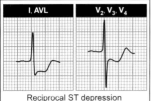

3° block with IJR

38

Acute Right Ventricle MI

(ST segment elevation in Lead: V_4R (MCL_4R). Q wave and inverted T wave may also be present) Accompanies Inferior MI in 30% of cases.

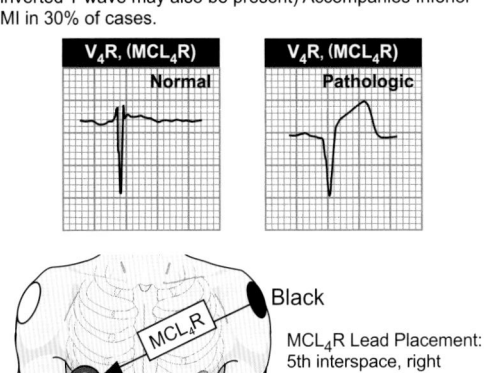

V_4R, (MCL_4R)	V_4R, (MCL_4R)
Normal	Pathologic

Black

MCL_4R Lead Placement: 5th interspace, right mid-clavicular line; monitor lead III.

Red

RCA is occluded. May cause: **AV block**, A-Fib, A-Flutter, right heart failure, JVD with clear lungs, **BP may drop if preload is reduced** (be cautious with morphine, NTG, furosemide). Treat hypotension with IV fluids, pacing.

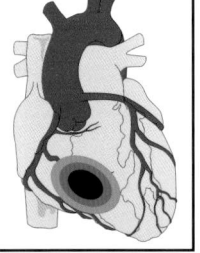

Acute Lateral MI

(ST segment elevation ≥0.5–1 mm in Leads: I, AVL, V_5, V_6.
Q waves and inverted T waves may also be present)

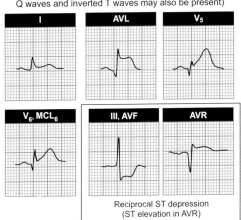

Reciprocal ST depression
(ST elevation in AVR)

NOTE: Lateral MI may be a component of a multiple site infarction, including anterior, inferior and/or posterior MI.

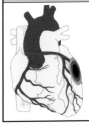

The circumflex branch of the left coronary artery is occluded. May cause: left ventricular dysfunction, **AV nodal block**.

Acute Posterior MI*

(ST segment depression with or without large R waves in Leads: V_1, V_2, V_3. Inverted T waves may also be present.)

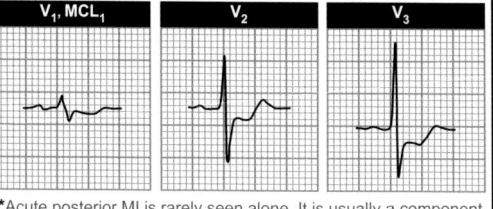

V_1, MCL_1	V_2	V_3

*Acute posterior MI is rarely seen alone. It is usually a component of a multiple site infarction, including inferior MI. If suspected, obtain posterior chest leads V_7–V_9 for diagnoses.

NOTE: RVH can also cause a large R wave in V_1. Rule out RVH first.

The right coronary artery or the circumflex branch of the left coronary artery is occluded. May cause **sinus arrest**.

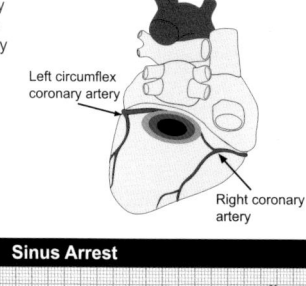

Left circumflex coronary artery

Right coronary artery

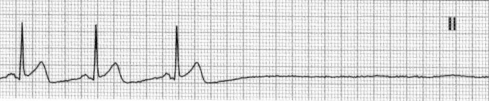

Sinus Arrest

II

Bundle Branch Block

Left BBB
(Notched/slurred R waves in I, or V_5, or V_6. Qs in V_1)

I, V_5, V_6

V_1, MCL_1

NOTE: If LBBB is present, do not attempt to diagnose AMI using only ECG criteria.

(QRS ≥ 0.12 second)

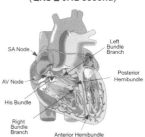

SA Node

AV Node

His Bundle

Right Bundle Branch

Left Bundle Branch

Posterior Hemibundle

Anterior Hemibundle

Right BBB
(Notched or two R waves in V_1 or V_2. Large S in I, V_5, V_6)

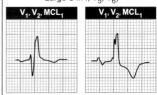

V_1, V_2, MCL_1

V_1, V_2, MCL_1

I, V_5, V_6

Electrolyte/Drug Effects

Hyperkalemia	Hypokalemia	Digitalis Effect
	All leads	
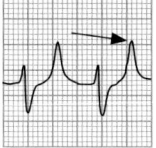		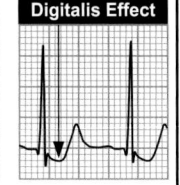
(Tall, peaked T waves; wide QRS and loss of P waves in extreme cases), patient is at risk for asystole, VF.	(Flat T wave, large U) **Patient is at risk for Torsades, VF, VT, hypokalemia exacerbates digitalis toxicity.**	(Depressed ST segments; asymmetrically inverted T.)

Torsades de Pointes

(2° anything that prolongs the QT interval: bradycardia, digitalis toxicity, quinidine, procainamide, disopyramide, phenothiazines, hypokalemia, hypomagnesemia, hypocalcemia, insecticide poisoning, subarachnoid hemorrhage, TCA OD.)

Medical Emergencies

Abbreviations Used In This Section

HX—History, Signs, and Symptoms
Key Symptoms and Findings (green text)
⊕—Prehospital Treatment (blue text with yellow background)
❖—Medical Emergency
Intermediate Procedures (blue italicized text)
Cautions—Contraindications or Precautions (red text)

General History For Most Patients

Events that led up to the chief complaint? Past Hx?
Medications? Allergies? Known diseases? Dyspnea (SOB)?
Previous trauma or surgery? Nausea and Vomiting (N/V)?
Fever (Fv)? MedicAlert®?

Pain Questions

- ❑ Location, radiation?
- ❑ Speed and time of onset, duration?
- ❑ Nature, what type of pain, tenderness?
- ❑ What makes it better or worse?
- ❑ Any associated symptoms?
- ❑ Ever had this pain before? What was it? Rate pain on a 1–10 scale, 10 being worst.

General Treatment For Most Patients

- Follow your local protocols at all times.
- Ensure ABCs (Airway, Breathing, Circulation).
- Treat life- or limb-threatening injuries immediately.
- Get vital signs (pulse, BP, respirations, effort, lung sounds).
- Monitor O_2 saturation; give O_2 as needed; protect airway.
- *Perform Intermediate procedures, as indicated (IV, ECG, etc.).*
- Transport as soon as practical.
- Monitor patient's condition en route.
- Reassure and comfort your patient.

Abdominal Pain—Common Causes

- ❖ **Epigastric**: AMI, gastroenteritis, ulcer, esophageal disease, heartburn
- ❖ **LUQ**: gastritis, pancreatitis, AMI, pneumonia
- ❖ **LLQ**: ruptured ectopic pregnancy, ovarian cyst, PID, kidney stones, diverticulitis, enteritis, abdominal abscess
- ❖ **RLQ**: appendicitis, ruptured ectopic pregnancy, enteritis, diverticulitis, PID, ovarian cyst, kidney stones, abdominal abscess, strangulated hernia
- ❖ **RUQ**: gall stones, hepatitis, liver disease, pancreatitis, appendicitis, perforated duodenal ulcer, AMI, pneumonia
- ❖ **Midline**: bladder infection, aortic aneurysm, uterine disease, intestinal disease, early appendicitis
- ❖ **Diffuse Pain**: pancreatitis, peritonitis, appendicitis, gastroenteritis, dissecting/rupturing aortic aneurysm, diabetes, ischemic bowel, sickle cell crisis

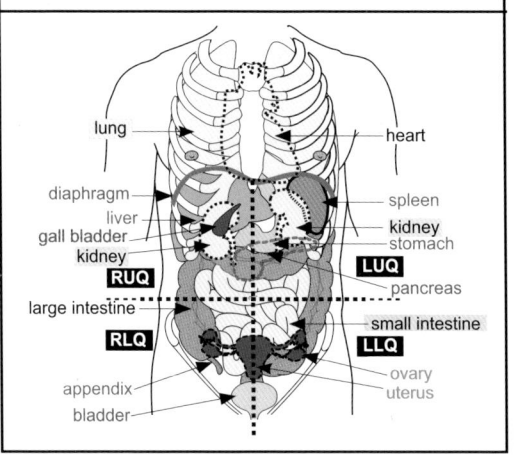

Abdominal Pain

HX—Ask **Pain Questions and General History**.
N/V? (color/quality of emesis)? Bowel movements, dysuria,
menstrual Hx, fever, postural hypotension, referred shoulder
pain? Is patient pregnant? Which trimester? Consider
ectopic pregnancy. Genitourinary, vaginal, or rectal bleeding/
discharge? Examine all 4 quadrants: abdominal tenderness,
guarding, rigidity, bowel tones present? Distension, pulsatile
mass? Record recent intake and GI habits. Vitals (sitting
and supine), Chemstrip®. Peripheral pulses equal?

➕—Position of comfort and NPO. Consider pulse oximetry.
O_2, IV (adjusted to vitals), consider ECG for epigastric pain.

CAUTION: Consider aortic aneurysm; ectopic pregnancy,
DKA. Epigastric abdominal pain may be cardiac.

- ❖ **Abdominal Aortic Aneurysm**: Severe abdominal pain,
  pulsatile mass, hypotension.
- ❖ **Acute MI**: Chest "pressure" or epigastric pain radiating
  to left arm or jaw, diaphoresis, N/V, SOB, pallor,
  dysrhythmias.
- ❖ **Appendicitls**: N/V, RLQ or periumbilical pain, fever, shock.
- ❖ **Bowel Obstruction**: N/V (fecal odor), localized pain.
- ❖ **Cholecystitis**: Acute onset RUQ pain and tenderness
  (may be referred to right shoulder/scapula)—may be
  related to high-fat meal. N/V, anorexia, fever. "Female,
  fat, 40."
- ❖ **Ectopic Pregnancy**: Missed period, pelvic pain,
  abnormal vaginal bleeding, dizziness.
- ❖ **Food Poisoning**: N/V, diffuse abdominal pain and
  cramping, diarrhea, fever, weakness, dizziness. Severe
  symptoms: descending paralysis, respiratory
  compromise.
- ❖ **Hepatic Failure**: Jaundice, confusion/coma, edema,
  bleeding and bruising, renal failure, fever, anorexia,
  dehydration.

Medical

- ❖ **Kidney Stone**: Constant or colicky severe flank pain, extreme restlessness, hematuria, N/V.
- ❖ **Pancreatitis**: Severe, "sharp," or "twisting" epigastric or LUQ pain radiating to back. N/V, diaphoresis, abdominal distention, signs of shock, fever.
- ❖ **Ulcer**: "Burning," epigastric pain, N/V, possible hematemesis, hypotension, decreased bowel sounds.

Notes

Abuse

✚—Remove the patient from the environment, transport to hospital. Report possible abuse to police, ED staff, protective services, and appropriate authorities. Call for police assistance, if needed, to protect the patient, and remove him/her from the scene. **Do not confront the alleged abuser.** Document your findings and any statements made by patient, family members, and others. Provide medical care, as needed. If sexual abuse is suspected, do not allow the patient to wash.

Non-Accidental Child Maltreatment

HX—Any unusual MOI, or one that does not match the child's injury/illness. Parents may accuse the child of hurting himself/herself, or may be vague/contradictory in providing history. There may be a delay in seeking medical care. The child may not cling to mother. Fracture in any child <2 years old; multiple injuries in various stages of healing, or on

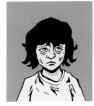

many parts of the body; obvious cigarette burns or wire marks; malnutrition; insect infestation, chronic skin infection, unkempt child. **Head injury is the leading cause of death of abused children**.

Intimate Partner Violence

HX—Repeated ED visits with injuries becoming more severe with each visit. Minimizing the seriousness or frequency of the injuries. Seeking treatment one or more days after the injuries. **Injuries that are not likely to have been caused by the accident reported**. Overprotective significant other who does not allow the patient to be alone with the health care professional. Fractures in different stages of healing, according to radiographic findings. History of child abuse to patient or partner.

Medical

Older Adult Maltreatment

HX—Fractures or bruises at various stages of healing. Unexplained bruises or cigarette burns on the torso or extremities. Soft tissue injuries from signs of restraint use. Head injuries. Malnourishment, listlessness, unexplained dehydration. Poor hygiene, inappropriate clothing. Decubitus ulcer, urine and feces on body and clothing. Unusual interaction between caregiver and patient.

✚—Remove the patient from the environment. Transport to hospital. Report possible abuse to police, ED staff, protective services, and appropriate authorities. Call for police assistance, if needed, to protect the patient and remove him/her from the scene. **Do not confront the alleged abuser.** Document your findings and any statements made by patient, family members, others. Provide medical care, as needed. If sexual abuse is suspected, do not allow the patient to wash.

Airway Obstruction

See "CHOKING."

Allergic Reaction

HX—Mild reaction (local swelling only) or serious systemic reaction (hives, pallor, bronchospasm, wheezing, upper airway obstruction with stridor, swelling of throat, hypotension). **If cardiac arrest, treat per ACLS.**

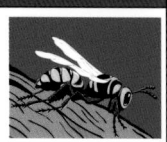

✚—If bee sting, remove stinger.
- For mild local reaction: wash area, apply cold pack.
- For serious reaction: secure airway, ventilate, O₂; large bore IV, titrate to BP >90; ECG; **Epinephrine: 1:1,000 SQ (Adult: 0.3 mL–0.5 mL; Pediatric: 0.01 mL/kg** [0.3 mL maximum]). Consider IV diphenhydramine and steroids for severe reactions.

Cautions—Epinephrine may cause arrhythmias or angina.

Altered Mental Status

Consider: Hypoglycemia, CVA/TIA, postical, alcohol, drugs, hypovolemia, head injury, hypothermia, HazMat, sepsis, shock, cardiogenic, vasovagal.

HX—Ask **Pain Questions and General History**. Time of onset: slow or fast? Seizure activity? Was patient sitting, standing, lying? Is patient pregnant (consider ectopic pregnancy)? Any recent illness or trauma? Current level of consciousness? Neurological status and psychological status? Any vomiting (bloody or coffee-ground)? Melena (black tarry stool)? Any signs of recent trauma?

➕—**General treatment**: Protect airway. Give O_2 as needed. Be prepared to assist ventilations. GCS <8? Intubate. Monitor ECG, vitals.

➕—**Cardiac: Support ABCs. Vitals, O_2**, treat per ACLS.

➕—**Coma**: (If multiple patients, suspect toxins—protect yourself!) Any odor at scene?—Consider HazMat. Were there any preceding symptoms or H/A? Past Hx: HTN, diabetes? Medications? Check scene for pill bottles or syringes and bring along. Get vitals, LOC and neuro findings, pupils. Any signs of trauma, drug abuse? Skin: color, temperature, rash, welts, facial or extremity asymmetry? MedicAlert® tag?

WARNING: Ensure your safety first, then the safety of patient and others.

- Secure airway, ventilate with 100% O_2, protect C-spine
- Start IV. Get Chemstrip®. Consider glucose, naloxone
- Monitor vital signs, O_2 saturation, and ECG

Cautions—Protect airway, suction as needed.

➕—**Sepsis/Infection**: O_2, IV, vitals. IV fluids for hypotension.

➕—**Syncope**: Position of comfort, O_2, IV, vitals, ECG. Consider IV fluids for hypotension.

Cautions—Syncope in middle-aged or elderly patients is often cardiac. Occult internal bleeding may cause syncope.

Childbirth (See also, OB/GYN Emergencies)

HX—Timing of contractions? Intensity? Does mother have urge to push or to move bowels? Has amniotic sac ruptured? Medications—any medical problems? Vital signs—check for:

- Vaginal bleeding or amniotic fluid; note color of fluid
- Crowning (means imminent delivery)
- Abnormal presentation (foot, arm, breech, cord, shoulder)

NOTE: Transport immediately if patient has had previous C-section, known multiple births, any abnormal presentation, excessive bleeding, or if pregnancy is not full-term and child will be premature.

➕—**Normal**: Control delivery using gloved hand to guide head, suction mouth and nose, deliver, keep infant level with perineum, clamp and cut cord 8"–10" from infant, **warm and dry infant**, stimulate infant by drying with towel, **make sure respirations are adequate**. Normal VS are: pulse: >120, respirations: >40, BP: 70, weight: 3.5 kg. Give baby 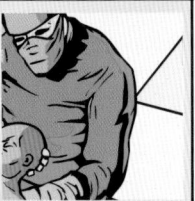 to mother to nurse at breast. Get APGAR scores at 1 and 5 minutes after birth. **If excessive post-partum bleeding, treat for shock, massage uterus to aid contraction, have mother nurse infant, start large bore IV**, consider oxytocin 10–40 units in 1,000 mL NS IV. Transport without waiting for placenta to deliver. Bring it with you to the hospital. Obtain mother's vital signs, O₂ saturation.

NOTE: Most births are normal—reassure mom and dad.

➕—**Breech**: Call OLMC. If head will not deliver, consider applying gentle pressure on mother's abdomen. Support legs and buttocks of baby; during contraction pull gently on baby. Encourage mother to pant, not push. If unsuccessful, insert your gloved fingers in vagina; deliver one shoulder, then the other. Do not pull on baby at this stage.

Deliver head by supporting baby's chest with your arms and hands. Place your fingers in vagina and find baby's mouth. Grasp the chin and apply gentle upward pressure to head and shoulders. Apply suprapubic pressure as well. If baby will not deliver, place fingers between baby's face and vaginal wall to create airway. **Rapid transport—patient may need emergency C-section.**

✚—**Cord Presents**: Call OLMC. Place mother in trendelenburg or knee-chest position, hold pressure on baby's head to relieve pressure on cord, check pulses in cord, keep cord moist with saline dressing, O_2, **rapid transport, start IV en route. Patient may require emergency C-section.**

✚—**Foot/Leg Presents**: Call OLMC. Support presenting part, place mother in trendelenburg or knee-chest position, O_2, **start IV**. Rapid transport.

✚—**Cord Around Neck**: **Unwrap cord from neck** and deliver normally, keep face clear, suction mouth and nose, etc.

✚—**Infant Not Breathing**: Stimulate with dry towel, rub back, flick soles of feet with finger. **Suction mouth and nose. Ventilate with BVM and 100% O_2** (this will revive most infants). **Begin chest compressions if HR <60.** If child does not respond, contact OLMC and reassess quality of ventilation efforts, lung sounds (pneumothorax? obstruction?) O_2 connected? **Intubate and ventilate.** Epinephrine 0.01 mg/kg IV/IO, or 0.1 mg/kg 1:1,000 ET; and IV fluids 10 mL/kg, glucose 2 mL/kg D25%W. **Rapid transport.** See Peds section, Pediatric Arrest.

Cautions—Failure to respond usually indicates hypoxia— **airway management is paramount in neonates.**

Medical

APGAR Scale

	0 points	1 point	2 points	1 Min	5 Min
Heart rate	Absent	<100	>100		
Resp. Effort	Absent	Slow, Irregular	Strong cry		
Muscle Tone	Flaccid	Some flex	Active motion		
Irritability	No response	Some	Vigorous		
Color	Blue, pale	Body: pink Extremities: Blue	Fully pink		
			TOTAL:		

Infants with scores of 7–10 usually require supportive care only. **A score of 4–6 indicates moderate depression**.

NOTE: Infants with scores of 3 or less require aggressive resuscitation.

Notes

Chest Pain

❖—Consider: **AMI, CHF, APE, pneumothorax, pneumonia, bronchitis, pulmonary embolus.**
HX—Ask **Pain Questions and General History**. Syncope, dizziness, weakness, diaphoresis? Fever, pallor? Dyspnea?
Past Hx: Chest trauma? Cardiac or respiratory problems, diabetes, high blood pressure, heart failure? Lung sounds, JVD? Peripheral or pulmonary edema? General appearance?

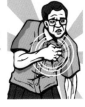

➕—Position of comfort, reassure patient, vitals, O_2, ECG, IV. Consider nitroglycerine for cardiac chest pain: 0.4 mg SL every 5 minutes (maximum: 3 doses). Consider aspirin for AMI.

IMPORTANT: Notify ED if your cardiac patient is a possible fibrinolytic candidate, and transport ASAP.

Cautions—Treat dysrhythmias according to ACLS.

❖ **Acute MI**: Severe, crushing chest pain, or substernal "pressure," radiating to the left arm, or jaw. N/V, SOB, diaphoresis, pallor, dysrhythmias, HTN or hypotension.
❖ **Aortic Dissection**: Sudden onset "tearing" chest or back pain, tachycardia, HTN or hypotension, diaphoresis, possible unequal pulses or unequal BP in extremities.
❖ **Cholecystitis**: Acute onset RUQ pain and tenderness (may be referred to right shoulder/scapula)—may be related to high-fat meal; N/V, anorexia, fever. "Female, fat, 40."
❖ **Hiatal Hernia**: Positional epigastric pain.
❖ **Musculo-Skeletal**: Pain on palpation, respiration. Obvious signs of trauma.
❖ **Pleurisy**: Pain on inspiration, fever, pleural friction rub.

- ❖ **Pneumonia**: Fever, shaking, chills, pleuritic chest pain, crackles, productive cough, tachycardia, diaphoresis.
- ❖ **Pulmonary Embolus**: Sudden onset SOB, cough, chest pain which is sharp and pleuritic, tachycardia, rapid respirations, O_2 sat <94%, apprehension, diaphoresis, hemoptysis, crackles.
- ❖ **Ulcer**: "Burning" epigastric pain, N/V, possible hematemesis, hypotension, decreased bowel sounds.

Notes

CPR—Adult, Child, or Infant

1. **Unresponsive?** (not breathing, or only gasping?)
2. **Call for assistance**—have someone get defibrillator/AED
3. **Check pulse within 10 seconds** (if present, give 1 breath every 5–6 seconds; check pulse every 2 minutes)— *if NO PULSE:*
4. **Position patient supine** on hard, flat surface
5. **Begin chest compression**s, 30:2, push hard and fast ≥100/minute, allow full chest recoil—minimize interruptions
6. **Open airway:** head-tilt/chin-lift, ventilate x2* (avoid excessive ventilations)
7. **Attach AED** to adult (and child >1 year old)

Shockable rhythm?

Yes ◀—————————————————————▶ **No**

Yes	**No**
8. **Shock x1**	8. **Resume CPR**
9. **Resume CPR**	**immediately** x2 minutes
immediately x2 minutes	9. **Initiate**
10. **Check rhythm**—	**ALS interventions**
if shockable:	10. **Check rhythm** every
11. **Shock x1;** resume CPR	2 minutes

 ◀—— lower half of sternum

head-tilt/chin-lift ——▶

CPR	Ratio	Rate	Depth	Check Pulse
Adult: 1 Person	30:2	100	>2"	Carotid
Adult: 2 Person	30:2	100	>2"	Carotid
Child: 1 Person	30:2	100	2"	Carotid
Child: 2 Person	15:2	100	2"	Carotid
Infant: 1 Person	30:2	100	1/3 cx	Brachial, Fem.
Infant: 2 Person	15:2	100	1/3 cx	Brachial, Fem.
Newborn: 2 Person	3:1	100	1/3 cx	Brachial, Fem.

*Adult—once an advanced airway is placed, ventilate at 8–10/minute.

Medical

Choking

For Responsive Choking Adult Or Child >1 Year

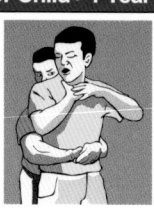

1. If patient cannot talk or has stridor, or cyanosis
2. **Perform Heimlich Maneuver** (use chest thrusts if patient is pregnant or obese), repeat until successful or patient is unconscious
3. **Begin CPR/call for assistance**
4. **Open airway; head-tilt/chin-lift** (look and remove object, if visible)
5. **Ventilate with two breaths**, if unable
6. **Reposition head; attempt to ventilate**, if unable
7. **Perform chest compressions (30:2)**
8. **Repeat: inspect mouth → remove object → ventilate → chest compressions** until successful
9. **Consider laryngoscopy and removal of object** by forceps, ET intubation, transtracheal ventilation, cricothyrotomy
10. If patient resumes breathing, place in the recovery position

For Unresponsive Choking Adult Or Child

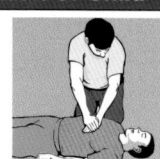

1. **Determine unresponsiveness**
2. **Call for assistance**
3. **Position patient supine** on hard, flat surface
4. **Open airway**—head-tilt/chin-lift (look and remove object if visible)
5. **Attempt to ventilate**, if unable
6. **Reposition head and chin, attempt to ventilate**, if unable
7. **Begin chest compressions (30:2)**
8. **Repeat: inspect mouth → remove object → ventilate → chest compressions** until successful
9. **Consider laryngoscopy and removal of object** by forceps, ET intubation, transtracheal ventilation, cricothyrotomy
10. If patient resumes breathing, place in the recovery position

For Choking Infant

1. **Confirm obstruction**: if infant can not make sounds, breathe, cry or is cyanotic
2. **Invert infant on arm**: support head by cupping face in hand; **perform 5 back slaps and 5 chest thrusts** until object is expelled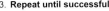
3. **Repeat until successful**
4. If patient becomes unconscious, **start CPR**
5. **Open airway, and ventilate x2**—if unable
6. **Reposition head and chin**, attempt to ventilate again
7. **Begin chest compressions (30:2)**
8. **Consider** laryngoscopy and removal of object by forceps, ET intubation, transtracheal ventilation, cricothyrotomy
9. If patient resumes breathing, place in the recovery position

Drowning and Near Drowning

HX—How long was patient submerged? Fresh or salt water? Cold water (<40°F)? Diving accident? **Immobilize spine**. Vitals, pulse oximetry, neurological status, GCS, crackles or pulmonary edema with respiratory distress?

✛—Open airway, suction, assist ventilations, start CPR. C-Spine: stabilize before removing patient from water. O_2, IV, monitor ECG. If hypothermic: use heated O_2 and follow hypothermia protocols. Conserve heat with blankets.

Cautions—All unconscious patients should have **C-spine immobilization**. All near-drowning patients should be transported. Many deteriorate later and develop pulmonary edema.

NOTE: Prepare for vomiting; intubate if unconscious.

Hyperglycemia

HX—Slow onset, excessive urination, thirst. When was insulin last taken? Abdominal cramps, N/V, mental status, high glucose on Chemstrip®, skin signs, dehydration? Respirations: deep and rapid? Breath odor: acetone, fruity?

✚—Secure airway, vital signs, O$_2$, large bore IV, fluid challenge (balanced salt solution). Monitor ECG.

Hypoglycemia/Insulin Shock

HX—Sudden onset, low blood glucose on Chemstrip®. Last insulin dose? Last meal? Mental status? Diaphoresis, H/A, blurred vision, dizziness, tachycardia, tremors, seizures?

✚—Support ABCs, O$_2$, vitals, IV. Give 50mL D50%W if patient is comatose (perform Chemstrip® before and after). Consider glucagon IM if unable to start IV. **Do not give oral glucose if airway is compromised.**

Cautions—Hypoglycemia can mimic a stroke or Intoxication. Seizures, coma, and confusion are common symptoms. **When in doubt about the diagnosis, give glucose IV or PO.**

HYPOGLYCEMIA	vs.	HYPERGLYCEMIA
Also known as	HYPOGLYCEMIA "Insulin Shock"	HYPERGLYCEMIA "DKA" "Ketoacidosis"
Incidence	More common	Less common
Blood sugar	Low (≤ 80 mg%)	High (≥180 mg%)
Onset	Rapid (minutes)	Gradual (days)
Skin	Moist, pale	Dry, warm
Respirations	Normal	Deep or rapid
Pulse	Normal or fast	Rapid, weak
Blood Pressure	Normal or high	Normal or low
Breath odor	Normal	Ketone/Acetone odor
Seizures	Common	Uncommon
Dehydration	No	Yes
Urine Output	Normal	Excessive
Thirst	Normal	Very Thirsty
Mental Status	Disoriented, Coma	Awake, weak, tired
Treatment	Glucose IV or PO	IV Fluids, Insulin, K$^+$
Recovery	Rapid (minutes)	Gradual (days)

Hyperthermia/Heat Stroke

HX—Onset? Exercise or drug (cocaine) induced? Vitals, temperature, skin: warm, dry?

✚—Remove from hot environment. Secure airway. Give O_2. Undress and begin cooling patient. Consider cold packs to groin, armpits. **Evaporation and convection measures work best** (but avoid causing shivering, as this may increase patient temperature). Start large bore IV. Consider fluid challenge. Monitor ECG. Reassess vital signs en route.

Cautions—Rapid cooling is key. Do not delay transport.

Hypothermia (See also, ACLS section, Hypothermia)

HX—Vital signs, mental status. Is patient cold? Shivering? Evidence of local injury?
Mild hypothermia: Shivering, ↑HR, ↑RR, lethargy, confusion.
Moderate hypothermia: ↓Respirations, ↓HR, rigidity, LOC, "J wave" on ECG.
Severe hypothermia: Coma, ↓BP, ↓HR, acidosis, VF, systole.

✚—Secure airway. Remove patient from cold environment **Give heated O_2**. A severely hypothermic patient may breathe slowly. Monitor ECG, large bore IV. **If cardiac arrest**, **start CPR** (see also, *ACLS section, Hypothermia*). Contact OLMC. Cut wet clothing off (do not pull off), wrap patient with blankets. Record vital signs, including temperature.

Cautions—Handle patient gently. Jostling can cause cardiac arrest. **If patient is not shivering**, **do not ambulate**. Stimulating the airway can cause cardiac arrest.

Medical

Infectious Diseases

Disease	Spread By	Risk To You
AIDS/HIV	IV/Sex/Blood products	↓Immune function, Pneumonias, Cancer
Anthrax	*Cutaneous:* contact with skin lesions	Infection = 25% mortality, but much lower if treated
	Ingestion: eating contaminated meat	Infection = high mortality, unless treated with antibiotics
	Pulmonary: inhaled spores	Infection = 95% mortality, but much lower if treated
C-diff	Secretions/ Excretions Hand to nose	Diarrhea, nausea, shock
Hepatitis A*	Fecal-oral	Acute hepatitis, jaundice
Hepatitis B*	IV/Sex/Birth/Blood	Acute and chronic hepatitis, cirrhosis, liver CA
Hepatitis C	Blood	Chronic hepatitis, cirrhosis, liver CA
Hepatitis D	IV/Sex/Birth	Chronic liver disease
Hepatitis E	Fecal-oral	↑Mortality to pregnant women and fetus
Herpes	Skin contact	Skin lesions, shingles
Influenza	Droplet/Airborne	Fever, pneumonia, prostration
MRSA	Secretions/ Excretions Hand to nose	Ulceration, tissue destruction
Meningitis*	Nasal secretions	Low risk to rescuer
Norovirus	Fecal to oral Hand to mouth	Diarrhea, nausea, vomiting
Tuberculosis	Sputum/cough/ Airborne	Cough, weight loss, lung damage

Universal Precautions

- ✔ Wear gloves for all patient contacts and for all contacts with body fluids.
- ✔ Wash hands after patient contact.
- ✔ Wear a mask for patients who are coughing or sneezing. Place a mask on the patient too.
- ✔ Wear eye shields or goggles when body fluids may splash.
- ✔ Wear gowns when needed.
- ✔ Wear utility gloves for cleaning equipment.
- ✔ Do not recap, cut, or bend needles.
- ✔ *Get vaccinated against hepatitis A, B, and Meningitis A, C, W, Y.

IMPORTANT: Report every exposure and get treatment immediately.

Notes

Medical

OB/GYN Emergencies

❖ **Abruptio Placenta:** Separation of placenta from uterine wall. Usually occurs >20 weeks gestation. Painful 3rd trimester vaginal bleeding (dark red), hypovolemic shock, hypotension, tachycardia, fetal distress, ↓FHT, ↑fundal height, pale skin, diaphoresis.

➕ —IV, O_2, rapid transport—patient may require emergency C-section.

❖ **Placenta Previa:** Placenta covers cervical os, can occur during 2nd and 3rd trimester. Painless bright red vaginal bleeding, possible hypotension, tachycardia.

➕ —O_2, IV, OB consult; if bleeding is heavy, rapid transport—patient may require C-section.

❖ **Preeclampsia/PIH:** (Pregnancy induced hypertension). HTN, H/A, proteinuria, edema of hands, feet, face and sacrum, weight gain, ↓urine output, visual disturbances, possible ↑liver enzymes, ↑neurologic reflexes, ↑chance of seizures, ↓FHT.

➕ —Transport quietly and gently, vitals; IV; treat HTN with labetalol, seizure prophylaxis with magnesium sulfate; OB consult, supportive care.

Physiologic Changes of Pregnancy

BP	Pulse	CO	ECG	Respirations	ABG	Blood Work	Other
↘	↑	↑	T Wave changes L II, aVF, aVL	↑Resp Rate ↑Tidal Volume ↓Vital Capacity ↓Functional residual capacity	↑pH ↑PaO₂ ↓PaCO₂ ↓HCO₃ Respiratory Alkalosis	↓HCT, ↑WBC ↑Fibrinogen ↑Clotting factors, Prone to DIC, ↑Blood Volume	↑N/V, aspiration ↑Injury: uterus, pelvis, bladder ↑Falls ↑Peripheral venous pressure

63

Maternal Cardiac Arrest

Activate Maternal Cardiac Arrest Team (document start time)
Consider and Treat Causes❖ (below)
Assess C-A-B, secure airway, give 100% O$_2$
⇩

Start CPR (hand placement higher on sternum than usual;
use continuous cricoid pressure for ventilations).
Defibrillate as usual—See *ACLS section, Adult Cardiac Arrest*
Give standard ACLS drugs and doses
If receiving IV/IO magnesium, **stop infusion and give
1 gm calcium chloride 10% (10 mL)** IV/IO *OR:*
3 gm calcium gluconate 10% (30 mL) IV/IO.
Start IV above the diaphragm—fluid bolus for hypovolemia

Experienced provider for advanced airway placement:
• may require smaller ET tube
• monitor for airway bleeding
• **preoxygenate to prevent hypoxia**
• RSI with cricoid pressure preferred
• choose sedative which will minimize hypotension

Monitor waveform capnography and CPR.
If PETCO$_2$ <15, improve CPR. ⇨
If obvious gravid uterus:
• Manually displace uterus to left to relieve
aortocaval compression
• Remove any internal and external fetal
monitors
• **Prepare for emergency cesarean
section if no ROSC in 4 minutes**

manual left uterine
displacement

• Goal: delivery within 5 minutes of
beginning CPR
• Continue maternal resuscitation during and after C-section

❖ Special Causes:

• Acidosis	• HTN/Eclampsia	• Placenta Abruption
• Amniotic fluid	• Hyper/	• Placenta Previa
embolus	Hypokalemia	• Sepsis
• Anesthetic effects	• Hypothermia	• Tension
• Bleeding	• Hypovolemia	Pneumothorax
• Cardiac disease	• Hypoxia	• Toxins
• Cardiac tamponade	• MI	• Uterine Atony
• DIC	• PE	

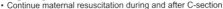

64

Organ and Tissue Donation

TISSUE	AGE	RESTRICTIONS
Bone	15–75	No IV drug use, no malignancy, no transmissible disease
Eyes	Any age	No systemic infection, no IV drug use, no transmissible disease
Heart valves	NB–55	No IV drug use, no malignancy, no transmissible disease
Organs	NB–70	Brain dead or potential to meet brain death, ventilator-dependent
Skin	15–75	No IV drug use, no malignancy, no transmissible disease

NOTE: There are very few contraindications to donation.

Psychiatric Emergencies

HX—Recent crisis? Emotional trauma, suicidal, changes in behavior, drug/alcohol abuse? Toxins, head injury, diabetes, seizure disorder, sepsis or other illness? Ask about suicidal feelings, intent; does patient have a plan? Make judgement about whether patient will act on plan. Vitals, pupil signs, mental status, oriented? Any odor on breath? MedicAlert®? Any signs of trauma?

IMPORTANT: Make sure scene is safe—protect yourself!

✚—Contact OLMC or psychiatric hospital. ABCs. Restrain patient as needed. If patient is suicidal, do not leave alone. Remove dangerous objects (weapons, pills, etc.). Transport in calm, quiet manner, if possible. Consider: O_2, IV, check blood sugar. If low, consider glucose PO or IV.

CAUTION: Always suspect hypoglycemia, and look for other medical causes: ETOH, drugs, sepsis, CVA, etc.

Respiratory Distress

HX—Ask **Pain Questions and General History**. Onset of event: was it slow or fast? **Fever? Cough? Is cough productive? Recent respiratory infection? Does patient smoke (how much)?** Record patient's medications. Assess severity of dyspnea (mild, moderate, severe) and tidal volume. Single word sentences? Is cyanosis present? **Level of consciousness? Lung sounds: any wheezing, crackles, rhonchi, diminished sounds? Vitals? Pulse oximetry.** Is patient exhausted? Candidate for intubation? **Upper airway obstruction (stridor, hoarseness, drooling, coughing)? Chest pain? Itching, hives? Numbness of mouth and hands? Signs of CHF: JVD, wet lung sounds (crackles), peripheral edema?**

✚ —**General treatment**: Position of comfort (usually upright). Give O_2 as needed. Be prepared to assist ventilations. Monitor ECG, vitals. Start IV, SaO_2, End-Tidal CO_2.

Cautions—High flow O_2 can depress respirations in a patient with COPD. Prepare to assist respirations.

❖ **Anaphylaxis**: See ALLERGIC REACTION

❖ **Asthma**: "Wheezes"

✚ —Consider nebulized bronchodilators, and/or epinephrine 1:1,000 SQ (0.3 mg–0.5 mg). Consider Atrovent, steroids.

❖ **COPD**: "Wheezes, rhonchi."

✚ —Consider nebulized bronchodilators. Consider Atrovent, steroids.

❖ **Pulmonary Edema**:

✚ —Consider nebulized bronchodilators, furosemide, sublingual nitroglycerine, morphine, and CPAP.

❖ **Tension Pneumothorax**:

✚ —Contact OLMC. Lift occlusive dressing, needle thoracentesis. **Rapid transport**.

Medical

Scene Safety

CAUTION: Wait until police secure the scene before entering: intimate partner violence, assault, any shooting or stabbing.

- ❑ As you approach, scan the area for hazards such as: hostile persons, dogs, uncontrolled traffic, spilled chemicals, gas, oil, down power lines
- ❑ Keep your exit routes open
- ❑ Any weapons present at the scene should be secured
- ❑ Wear protective gear. Call for more resources if needed

Crime Scene

IMPORTANT: Consider the safety of your crew first. Consider staging out of sight until scene is secure.

Access and Treatment

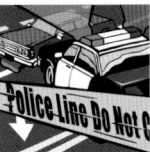

1. Consult with police regarding best access.
2. Make a mental note of physical and weather conditions.
3. Do not park your vehicle over visible tire tracks.
4. To avoid destroying evidence, select a single route to and from the victim.
5. Limit the number of personnel allowed on scene.
6. Be conscious of any statements made.
7. Do not cut through any holes in patients' clothing.
8. Place victim on a clean sheet for transport. After transport, obtain the sheet, fold it onto itself, and give to the police.
9. When moving the victim, it is important to note:
   - Location of furniture prior to moving
   - Position of victim prior to moving
   - Status of clothing
   - Location of any weapons or other articles
   - Name of personnel who moved items
10. Consult with police regarding whether to pick up medical debris left over from treatment.
11. Write a detailed report regarding your crews actions.

Seizures

❖ Consider **epilepsy, hypoxia, CVA, cardiac origin, ETOH/drug use/withdrawal, hypoglycemia, pregnancy, hyperthermia, infection,** or **metabolic cause.**

HX—Type (generalized or partial), onset, length, seizure history or meds? Compliance? Recent head trauma? What was patient doing before seizure? Did patient fall? Bite tongue? Dysrhythmias? Incontinent? Is seizure drug-induced (antidepressant cocaine)? MedicAlert®? Level of consciousness? Head or oral trauma? Focal neurologic signs? H/A? Respiratory status?

⊞— **Generalized**: Keep airway open, consider NPA (do not use EOA/EGTA), O₂, suction, IV, test CBG, consider IV glucose, benzodiazepines as needed, transport on side. Monitor ECG, vitals.

⊞—**Partial**: Do not grab patient; may lead to violent reaction. Block patient's access to doors, windows, etc. Direct, do not restrain. Use calm reassurance. Establish LOC. Monitor recovery.

⊞—**Patient having seizure who has VNS implant**: Pass patient's wrist magnet over VNS (Vagus Nerve Stimulator) on slow 3-second count. Implant usually in upper left chest. Repeat every 3–5 minutes, maximum of 3 times. If VNS does not stop seizure, treat per **Generalized** guidelines above.

Cautions—Seizure in water can lead to APE. Transport for evaluation. Restrain patient only to prevent injury—protect patient's head. Do not force anything into the mouth. Always check for a pulse after seizure stops. Most seizures are self-limiting, lasting less than 1–2 minutes.

NOTE: Not all patients having a seizure need transport.

Shock

HX—Ask **Pain Questions and General History**. Onset? Associated symptoms: hives, edema, thirst, weakness, dyspnea, chest pain, dizziness when upright, abdominal pain? Trauma? Bloody vomitus or stools? Delayed capillary refill? Tachypnea? Syncope? N/V? Mental status: confusion, restlessness? Tachycardia, hypotension? Skin: pale, sweaty, cool. Signs of pump failure: JVD while upright, crackles, peripheral edema.

✚—Stop hemorrhage, if any. Apply direct pressure to wound. Consider pressure point or tourniquet. Place patient supine, O_2 high flow, assist ventilations as needed, Start large bore IV. **Do not delay transport to start IV.** (Consider intraosseous infusion if unable to start IV.) Prevent heat loss. Try to determine the type of shock (hypovolemic, cardiogenic, obstructive, distributive, etc.). **If trauma, enter patient in Trauma System.** Assess lung sounds. Monitor ECG, O_2 sat, vitals, level of consciousness.

Cautions—Check lung sounds for crackles before giving IV fluids and after each bolus.

Notes

Stroke/CVA

HX—New neuro symptoms <24 hours? Ambulatory at baseline? Preceding symptoms: headache, confusion, seizure, dizziness, loss of balance or coordination, trouble walking, sudden onset of numbness or weakness of the face, arm, or leg (especially on one side of the body), trouble speaking or seeing in one or both eyes? **Past HX**— HTN, Diabetes, seizure? **Findings**: Age >45 years, LOC, GCS, patient aware of name? MedicAlert® tag? CBG >60 and <400, pupils, vitals, meds? Neuro: Facial droop-smile/ grimice, slurred speech, difficulty understanding, hand grips, arm or leg drift, weakness, or paralysis?

✚—Airway, O₂, suction and assist ventilations as needed. IV, GCS, check blood glucose and give IV glucose, if hypoglycemic. Vitals, ECG (CVA may be 2° to cardiac event).

Patient may be candidate for fibrinolysis. Consider rapid transport.

Brain Areas

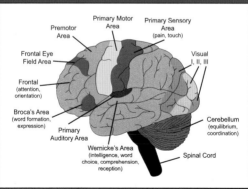

Premotor Area

Primary Motor Area

Primary Sensory Area (pain, touch)

Frontal Eye Field Area

Visual I, II, III

Frontal (attention, orientation)

Broca's Area (word formation, expression)

Cerebellum (equilibrium, coordination)

Primary Auditory Area

Wernicke's Area (intelligence, word choice, comprehension, reception)

Spinal Cord

Medical

Posturing

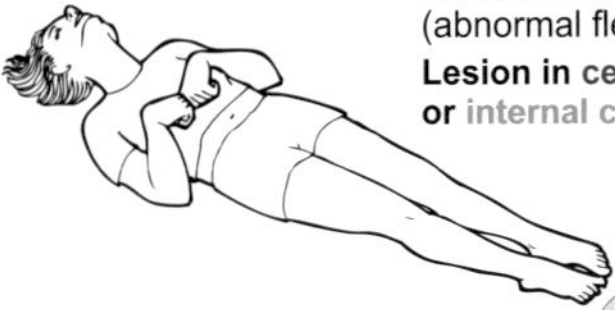

Decorticate:
(abnormal flexion)
Lesion in cerebral hemispheres
or internal capsule

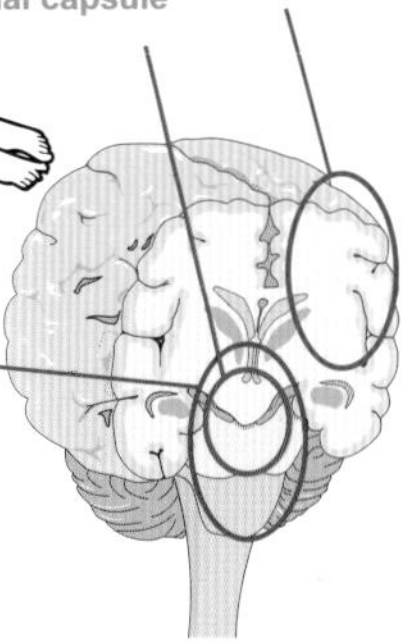

Decerebrate:
(abnormal extension)
Lesion midbrian, brain stem
or pons

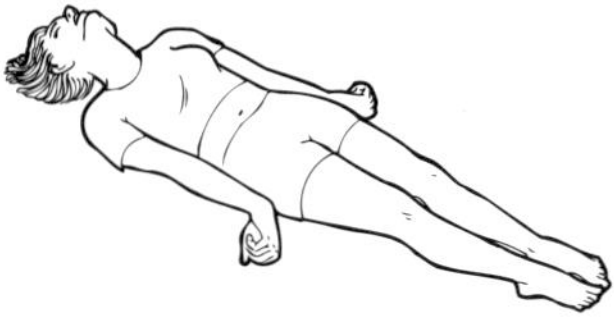

Pupil Gauge (in mm)

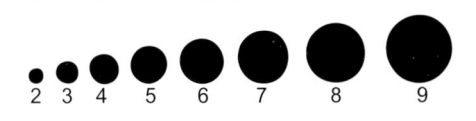

2 3 4 5 6 7 8 9

Fibrinolytic Checklist for Ischemic Stroke

All the "YES" boxes and all the "NO" boxes must be checked before fibrinolytic therapy can be given.

INCLUSION CRITERIA (all must be YES)
- ❑ Age 18 years or older
- ❑ Clinical Dx: ischemic stroke causing measurable neuro deficit
- ❑ Time of symptom onset will be <4.5* hours before fibrinolytic treatment begins (*<3 hours if any: >80 years old, severe stroke [NIHSS >25], on oral anticoagulant, Hx diabetes + prior ischemic stroke)

EXCLUSION CRITERIA (all must be NO)
- ❑ Prior stroke or head injury within the past 3 months
- ❑ Intracranial hemorrhage on noncontrast CT
- ❑ Clinical suspicion subarachnoid bleed, even with normal CT
- ❑ Arterial puncture within 7 days at a noncompressible site
- ❑ Multilobar infarction on CT >1/3 cerebral hemisphere
- ❑ Uncontrolled HTN: systolic BP >185 mm Hg or diastolic BP >110 mm Hg
- ❑ Evidence of active hemorrhage on exam
- ❑ Blood glucose <50 mg/dL (2.7 mmol/L)
- ❑ Hx: previous intracranial bleed, AV malformation, aneurysm, or neoplasm
- ❑ Active internal bleeding or acute trauma (fracture)
- ❑ Acute bleeding diathesis, including but not limited to:
  - ❑ Platelet count <100,000/mm^3
  - ❑ Patient has received heparin within 48 hours and had an elevated aPTT (greater than upper limit of normal for lab)
  - ❑ Current use of anticoagulant (e.g., warfarin sodium) with elevated prothrombin time >15 seconds, or INR >1.7

RELATIVE CONTRAINDICATIONS (weigh risks vs. benefits)
- ❑ Only minor or rapidly improving stroke symptoms
- ❑ Within 14 days of major surgery or serious trauma
- ❑ Within 21 days of GI or urinary tract hemorrhage
- ❑ Recent acute MI within 3 months
- ❑ Witnessed seizure at stroke onset, with postictal impairments

Los Angeles Prehospital Stroke Screen (LAPSS)

Screening Criteria:

1. Age over 45 years	❏ Yes ❏ No
2. No prior history of seizure disorder	❏ Yes ❏ No
3. New neurologic symptoms in last 24 hours	❏ Yes ❏ No
4. Patient was ambulatory prior to event	❏ Yes ❏ No
5. Blood glucose between 60–400	❏ Yes ❏ No
6. Exam (below) reveals only unilateral weakness	❏ Yes ❏ No

Exam: look for obvious asymmetry

	Normal	Right		Left	
Facial smile/grimace		Droop		Droop	
Grip		Weak grip		Weak grip	
		No grip		No grip	
Arm weakness		Drifts down		Drifts down	
		Falls rapidly		Falls rapidly	

7. If "Yes" to all items above, the LAPSS screening criteria are met: **Notify receiving hospital with "code stroke."**

NOTE: The patient may still be experiencing a stroke even if LAPSS criteria are not met.

Cincinnati Prehospital Stroke Scale

Symptoms	Normal	Abnormal
Facial droop	Both sides of face move equally	One side of face does not move as well as other side
Arm drift	Both arms move equally or not at all	One arm drifts compared to the other
Speech	Patient uses correct words with no slurring	Slurred or inappropriate words or mute

NOTE: Any abnormal finding suggests potential stroke.

Vaginal Bleeding (See also, OB/GYN Emergencies)

❖—Consider: **Miscarriage**, **ectopic pregnancy**, also **CA**, **trauma**.

HX—Ask **Pain Questions and General History**. Cramping? Clots, tissue fragments (bring to ER), dizziness, weakness, thirst (painless bleeding with pregnancy suggests placenta previa). Duration, amount; last menstrual period (normal or irregular)? If patient is pregnant: due date? **Past HX**— Bleeding problems, pregnancies, medications? Vitals and orthostatic change? Fever? Evidence of blood loss, signs of shock? Vasoconstriction, sweating, altered mental status.

✚—**General Treatment**: O_2, IV large bore, titrated to vitals, assess vitals, O_2 saturation, ECG.

Cautions—If miscarriage is suspected, field vaginal exam is generally not indicated.

✚—**Postpartum Bleeding**: Treat for shock, massage uterus to aid contraction, have mother nurse infant, start large bore IV, transport without waiting for placenta to deliver. Bring it with you to the hospital. Get vital signs.

✚—**Abruptio Placenta**: Painful 3rd trimester bleeding. Look for hypovolemic shock, give O_2, start IV. **Rapid transport**.

✚—**Placenta Previa**: Painless 3rd trimester bleeding. Start IV, O_2. **Rapid transport**.

Medical

Poisons and Overdoses

NOTE: This section is not a comprehensive list of of all drugs, poisons, side effects, cautions, or treatments. Before administering any treatments, consult your Poison Center, the product label or insert, your protocols, and/or your On-Line Medical Resource.

Abbreviations Used In This Section

AKA—Common brand®, ™, and "street names"
SE—Common toxic side effects (green text)
Cautions—Primary cautions (red text)
RX—Prehospital care (blue text)

Acids   • *Caustics*

AKA—Rust remover, metal polish.
SE—Pain, GI tract chemical burns, lip burns, vomiting.
RX—Give milk or water, milk of magnesia, egg white, prevent aspiration. Transport patient in sitting position, if possible.
Cautions—Do not induce vomiting.

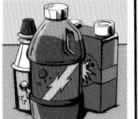

Acetaminophen   • *Analgesic*

AKA—Tylenol®, APAP.
SE—There may be no symptoms, but acetaminophen is toxic to the liver. N/V, anorexia, RUQ pain, pallor, diaphoresis.
RX—ABCs, O_2, IV, ECG, fluids for hypotension. Activated charcoal 1 gm/kg PO or by NG tube, if given within 4 hours of ingestion. Acetylcysteine may be given in ED.

Alkalis • Caustics

AKA—Drano®, drain and oven cleaners, bleach.
SE—Pain, GI tract chemical burns, lip burns, vomiting.
RX—Give milk or water, prevent aspiration. Transport patient in sitting position, if possible.
Cautions—Do not induce vomiting.

Amphetamines/Stimulants • Stimulant

AKA—Methamphetamine, "speed," "crank."
SE—Anxiety, ↑HR, arrhythmias, diaphoresis, seizure, N/V, H/A, CVA, HTN, hyperthermia, dilated pupils, psychosis, suicidal.
RX—ABCs, O₂, IV fluids for hypotension. Activated charcoal 50–100 gm orally. Maintain normal body temp. Benzodiazepine as adjunct.
Cautions—Protect yourself against the violent patient.

Antidepressants (TCA) • Mood Elevators

AKA—Norpramin®, Sinequan®, amitriptyline.
SE—Hypotension, PVCs, cardiac arrhythmias, QRS complex widening, seizures, coma, death.
RX—ABCs, O₂, IV, ECG, IV fluids, 1 mEq/kg NaHCO₃ IV, intubate and ventilate.
Cautions—Onset of coma and seizures can be sudden. Do not induce vomiting.

Aspirin • Analgesic

AKA—Bayer®, ASA, salicylates.
SE—GI bleeding, N/V, LUQ pain, pallor, diaphoresis, shock, tinnitus, ↑RR.
RX—ABCs, O₂, IV, ECG, fluids for hypotension. Activated charcoal 1 gm/kg PO.

76

Barbiturates/Sedatives · *Hypnotic*

AKA—Phenobarbital, "barbs," "downers."
SE—Weakness, drowsiness, respiratory depression, apnea, coma, hypotension, bradycardia, hypothermia, APE, death.
RX—ABCs, O₂, ventilate, IV fluids for hypotension.
Cautions—Protect the patient's airway.

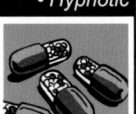

Carbon Monoxide · *Odorless Toxic Gas*

Causes—Any source of incomplete combustion, such as: car exhaust, fire suppression, and stoves.
SE—H/A, dizziness, DOE, fatigue, tachycardia, visual disturbances, hallucinations, cherry red skin color, ↓respirations, N/V, cyanosis, altered mental status, coma, blindness, hearing loss, convulsions.
RX—Remove patient from toxic environment, ABCs, 100% O₂ (check blood glucose), transport. Hyperbaric treatment in severe cases.
Cautions—O₂ sat monitor can give false high reading with CO exposure.

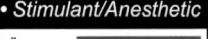

WARNING: Protect yourself from exposure!

Cocaine · *Stimulant/Anesthetic*

AKA—"Coke," "snow," "flake," "crack."
SE—H/A, N/V, ↓RR, agitation, ↑HR, arrhythmias, chest pain, vasoconstriction, AMI, HTN, seizure, vertigo, euphoria, paranoia, vomiting, hyperthermia, tremors, paralysis, coma, dilated pupils, bradycardia, death, APE with IV use.
RX—ABCs, O₂, IV, ET intubation. Consider: benzodiazepine for seizures, lidocaine for PVCs, nitrates, and phentolamine for AMI. Control HTN. Monitor VS and core temp: cool patient if hyperthermic. Minimize sensory stimulation. Consider activated charcoal for oral cocaine ingestion.
Cautions—Protect yourself from the violent patient. A "speedball" is cocaine + heroin. Do not give beta blockers.

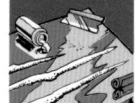

Ecstasy/MDMA • *Stimulant/Hallucinogen*

AKA—"XTC," "X," "love drug," "MDMA," "Empathy."
SE—Euphoria, hallucinations, agitation, teeth grinding (use of pacifiers), nausea, hyperthermia, sweating, HTN, tachycardia, renal and heart failure, dilated pupils, seizures, rhabdomyolysis, DIC, APE, CVA, coma, electrolyte imbalance.
RX—ABCs, O$_2$, vitals, ECG, IV, cool patient if hyperthermic, intubate if unconscious, benzodiazepine for seizure and bicarb for myoglobinurea.
Cautions—Do not give beta blockers.

GHB (Gamma-Hydroxybutyrate) • *Depressant*

AKA—"G," "easy lay," "liquid X," "Blue Nitro."
SE—Euphoria, sedation, dizziness, myoclonic jerking, N/V, H/A, coma, bradycardia, apnea.
RX—ABCs, manage airway, ventilate.
Cautions—A common "date rape" drug.

Hallucinogens • *Alter Perception*

AKA—LSD, psilocybin mushrooms.
SE—Anxiety, hallucinations, panic, disorientation, N/V.
RX—Calm and reassure the patient. Be supportive.
Cautions—Watch for violent and unexpected behavior.

Hydrocarbons • *Fuels, Oils*

AKA—Gasoline, oil, petroleum products.
SE—Breath odor, SOB, seizures, APE, coma, bronchospasm.
RX—ABCs, O$_2$, gastric lavage.
Cautions—Do not induce vomiting.

Opiates • *Narcotic Analgesic*

AKA—Dilaudid®, heroin, morphine, codeine, fentanyl.
SE—↓Respirations, apnea, ↓BP, coma, bradycardia, pinpoint pupils, vomiting, diaphoresis.
RX—ABCs, O₂, ventilate, intubate, IV fluids for hypotension, naloxone 2 mg IV/IO, IM, SQ, ET, IL.
Cautions—Consider other concurrent overdoses.

Organophosphates • *Insecticides*

AKA—Malathion®, Diazinon®.
SE—SLUDGE (Salivation, Lacrimation, Urination, Defecation, G-I, Emesis), pinpoint pupils, weakness, bradycardia, sweating, N/V, diarrhea, dyspnea.

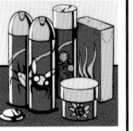

RX—Extricate patient, ABCs. O₂, Atropine 1–5 mg IV/IO, IM double doses every 5 minutes until sludge goes away. Start at 2 mg IV/IO, IM for moderate signs and symptoms.
Peds—*0.05 mg/kg, every five minutes, until vital signs improve.*
Cautions—Protect yourself first! Do not become contaminated.

PCP—Phencyclidine • *Tranquilizer*

AKA—"Peace Pill," "angel dust," "horse tranquilizer."
SE—Nystagmus, disorientation, HTN, hallucinations, catatonia, sedation, paralysis, stupor, mania, tachycardia, dilated pupils, status epilepticus.

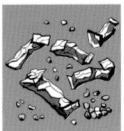

RX—ABCs, O₂, vitals, IV, ECG. Consider benzodiazepines.
Cautions—Protect yourself against violent patient. Examine patient for trauma which may have occurred due to anesthetic effect of PCP.

Tranquilizers (major) • *Antipsychotic*

AKA—Haldol®, Navane®, Thorazine®, Compazine®.

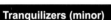

SE—EPS, dystonias, painful muscle spasms, respiratory depression, hypotension, torsades de pointes.

RX—Diphenhydramine 25–50 mg IV or deep IM for EPS. ABCs, O$_2$, vitals, ECG. Consider activated charcoal 50–100 gm orally. IV fluids for hypotension. Consider intubation for the unconscious patient.
Cautions—Protect the patient's airway.

Tranquilizers (minor) • *Anxiolytics*

AKA—Valium®, Xanax®, diazepam, midazolam.

SE—Sedation, weakness, dizziness, tachycardia, hypotension, hypothermia, (↓respirations with IV use).

RX—ABCs, monitor vitals; Flumazenil IV if no seizure history.
Cautions—Coma usually means some other substance or cause is also involved. OD is almost always in combination with other drugs. Protect the patient's airway.

Emergency Medications

NOTE: This section is not a complete or comprehensive list of all medications. For complete information, please consult the drug product insert, or an appropriate medical resource.

Abbreviations Used In This Section

RX—Primary indications (black text)
Contra—Primary contraindications (red text)
Dosages—(blue/bold text)
SE—Common side effects (green text)
• *Drug Type*—for medications (italic text)
Peds—Pediatric doses (black italic text)

Activated Charcoal • *Adsorbent*

RX—**Poisoning/Overdose: 1 gm/kg PO or by NG tube.**
(Mix with water to make a slurry.)
Contra—**Contact Poison Center for more advice.**
SE—Constipation, black stools, diarrhea.
Peds—1 gm/kg.

Adenosine (Adenocard®) • *Antiarrhythmic*

RX—**PSVT: 6 mg (2 mL) IV rapidly over 1–3 seconds**
(flush with 20 mL NS bolus; elevate IV arm). If no effect in
1–2 minutes, **give 12 mg over 1–3 seconds. May repeat
12 mg** bolus one more time.
Contra—Second degree or third degree AV block, VT, sick
sinus syndrome.
SE—Transient dysrhythmias, facial flushing, dyspnea, chest
pressure, ↓HR, ↓BP, H/A, nausea, bronchospasm.

NOTE: Adenosine is blocked by the ophyllines; but potentiated
by dipyridamole, carbamazepine.

Peds—0.1–0.2 mg/kg IV rapidly, IO up to 6 mg. May double
dose if no effect. Maximum: 12 mg/dose.*

Albuterol 0.5% (Ventolin®)   • *Bronchodilator*

RX—Bronchospasm 2° COPD, Asthma: 2.5 mg mixed in 3 mL saline in nebulizer.
Contra—Tachydysrhythmias, HTN, hypokalemia.
SE—Tachydysrhythmias, anxiety, N/V.
Peds—2.5 mg nebulized in 3 mL saline.

Alteplase (Activase® t-PA)   • *Fibrinolytic*

RX—Acute MI (<12 hours old): 100 mg IV over 3 hours.
Mix 100 mg in 100 mL sterile water for 1 mg/mL.
Accelerated 1.5-hour infusion:
• Administer **15 mg IV bolus** (15 mL) **over 2 minutes**
• Then give **0.75 mg/kg** (max: **50 mg**) over next 30 minutes
• Followed by **0.5 mg/kg** (max: **35 mg**) over next hour

RX—Acute Ischemic Stroke (<3 hours old): 0.9 mg/kg IV (maximum: **90 mg**) **over 1 hour.**
• Give 10% of the total dose as an IV bolus over 1 minute
• Then give the remaining 90% over the next hour

RX—Acute Pulmonary Embolism: 100 mg IV over 2 hours.

Contra—Any within 3 months: stroke, AV malformation, neoplasm, recent trauma, aneurysm, recent surgery. Active internal bleeding within 21 days; major surgery or trauma within 14 days, aortic dissection, severe HTN, known bleeding disorders, prolonged CPR with thoracic trauma, LP within 7 days, arterial puncture at a non-compressible site. See *ACLS section, Stemi Fibrinolytic Protocol,* for more contraindications.
SE—Reperfusion dysrhythmias, bleeding, shock.

Amiodarone (Cordarone®) • Antiarrhythmic

RX—Cardiac Arrest VF/VT: 300 mg IVP. May repeat 150 mg IVP every 3–5 minutes. Maximum: 2,200 mg/24 hours.

RX—Stable Wide Complex Tachycardia:

Rapid infusion:
150 mg IV over 10 minutes. May repeat 150 mg IVP every 10 minutes (mix 150 mg in 100 mL; run at 10 mL/minute or **600 microdrop/minute**). Maximum 2,200 mg/24 hours.

Slow infusion:
360 mg IV over 6 hours (mix 1,000 mg in 500 mL; run at 30 mL/hour or **30 microdrop/minute**).

Maintenance infusion:
540 mg IV over 18 hours (mix 1,000 mg in 500 mL; run at 15 mL/hour or **15 microdrop/minute**).

Contra—Cardiogenic shock, bradycardia, 2°, 3° block; do not use with drugs that prolong QT interval.
SE—Vasodilation, ↓BP, ↓HR, AV block, hepatotoxicity, ↑QTc, VF, VT, 40 day half-life.
Peds—5 mg/kg IV/IO.

Amyl Nitrite • Cyanide Antidote

RX—Cyanide Poisoning: Administer vapors from crushed inhalant for 30 seconds, then administer oxygen for 30 seconds, repeat continuously. Consider following with sodium nitrite and sodium thiosulfate.
SE—Hypotension, H/A, nausea.

Aspirin (ASA) • Antiplatelet

RX—Acute Myocardial Infarction: 160–325 mg PO (2–4 chewable children's aspirin tablets).
Contra—Allergy. Use caution with: asthma, ulcers, GI bleeding, other bleeding disorders.
SE—GI bleeding.

Atenolol (Tenormin®)   • *Beta Blocker*

RX—VT, VF, Atrial Fib, Atrial Flutter, PSVT, HTN.

RX—Myocardial Salvage for:
- Acute Anterior MI with HTN and Tachycardia
- Large MI <6 hours old
- Refractory Chest Pain or Tachycardia 2° excess sympathetic tone

5 mg IV slowly over 5 minutes. Wait 10 minutes. Then give another 5 mg IV slowly over 5 minutes. If tolerated well, in 10 minutes, give 50 mg, PO dose, titrate to effect.
Contra—CHF, APE, bronchospasm, Hx asthma, ↓HR, 2° or 3° heart block, cardiogenic shock, ↓BP.
SE—↓BP, CHF, bronchospasm, ↓HR, chest pain, H/A, N/V.

NOTE: Calcium blockers may exacerbate side effects.

Atropine Sulfate   • *Vagolytic*

RX—Symptomatic Bradycardia: 0.5–1 mg IVP every 3–5 minutes; up to 0.04 mg/kg total dose, or 3 mg.

RX—Organophosphate or Carbamate Insecticide Poisoning: 1–5 mg IV/IO, IM double doses every 5 minutes until sludge goes away. Start at 2 mg IV/IO, IM for moderate signs and symptoms.
Peds—0.05 mg/kg, every five minutes, until vital signs improve.

RX—Asthma: 0.4–2 mg nebulized in 3 mL saline.
RX—RSI (pediatric): 0.02 mg/kg. Minimum 0.1 mg

Contra—Tachycardia, glaucoma.
SE—Dilated pupils, ↑HR, VT, VF, H/A, dry mouth.

Calcium Chloride 10%   • *Electrolyte*

RX—Calcium Blocker Toxicity, Hypocalcemia with Tetany, Hyperkalemia, Hypermagnesemia: 500–1,000 mg IV over 5–10 minutes.
Contra—VF, digitalis toxicity, hypercalcemia.
SE—↓HR, ↓BP, VF, coronary and cerebral artery spasm, N/V; extravasation causes necrosis.

NOTE: Precipitates with $NaHCO_3$ in IV bag/tubing.

Peds—10–20 mg/kg (0.1–0.2 mL/kg) IV/IO slowly.

Dexamethasone (Decadron®) • Anti-inflammatory

RX—Cerebral Edema, Anaphylaxis, COPD, Spinal Trauma:
10–100 mg IV.
Contra—Uncontrolled infections, TB, ulcers.
Peds—0.25–1 mg/kg IV/IO, IM.

Dextrose 50% • Nutrient

RX—Coma, Hypoglycemia: 25 gm (50 mL) IV.
SE—Tissue necrosis if extravasation occurs.
Contra—Intracerebral bleeding, hemorrhagic CVA.

Diazepam (Valium®) • Anticonvulsant/Sedative

RX—Status Epilepticus: 5–10 mg IV slowly.

RX—Sedation: 5–15 mg IV slowly. (Rectal diazepam:
0.5 mg/kg via 2" rectal catheter. Flush with 2–3 mL of air
after administration.)
Contra—Head injury, ↓BP, acute narrow angle glaucoma.
SE—↓Respirations, ↓BP, drowsiness, venous irritation.

NOTE: Overdose may be reversed with flumazenil.

Diphenhydramine (Benadryl®) • Antihistamine

RX—Allergic Reaction, EPS: 25–50 mg IV, or deep IM.
Contra—Asthma, pregnant or lactating females.
SE—Sedation, blurred vision, anticholinergic effects.
Peds—1–2 mg/kg IV/IO slowly, or IM.

Diltiazem (Cardizem®) • Antiarrhythmic

RX—PSVT, Rapid Atrial Fibrillation, Atrial Flutter:
0.25 mg/kg IV/IO slowly over 2 minutes; if no effect in
15 minutes; **0.35 mg/kg IV/IO slowly over 2 minutes.** Drip:
10–15 mg/hour (5 mg/hour for some patients).

Diltiazem (5mg/mL) Bolus Doses in mL	Patient weight in kg					
	50	60	70	80	90	100
1st dose: 0.25 mg/kg →	2.5 mL	3 mL	3.5 mL	4 mL	4.5 mL	5 mL
2nd dose: 0.35 mg/kg →	3.5 mL	4.2 mL	4.9 mL	5.6 mL	6.3 mL	7 mL

[for drip: mix 125 mg (25 mL) in 100 mL IV solution (1 mg/mL) & run at:]

Diltiazem Drip	mg/hour →	5 mg	10 mg	15 mg
	microdrops/minute →	5 gtt	10 gtt	15 gtt

Contra—Second degree or third degree block, ↓BP, sick sinus syndrome, VT; WPW or short PR syndrome with atrial fib or atrial flutter. Do not give with oral beta blockers. Do not give with furosemide in same IV line (flush line first).
SE—Hypotension, bradycardia, H/A, N/V, CHF, dizziness, weakness. Diltiazem ↑serum digoxin levels.

Dopamine (Intropin®)   • *Inotrope*

RX—**Hypotension, Bradycardia**: 2–20 mcg/kg/minute.

> Renal Dose: 2–5 mcg/kg/minute
> Inotropic Dose: 5–10 mcg/kg/minute
> Pressor Dose: >10 mcg/kg/minute

Mix 400 mg in 250 mL D5W (1,600 mcg/mL) and run at:

mcg/kg/ min	Patient weight in kg											
	2.5	5	10	20	30	40	50	60	70	80	90	100
2 mcg	–	–	–	1.5	2	3	4	5	5	6	7	8
5 mcg	–	1	2	4	6	8	9	11	13	15	17	19
10 mcg	1	2	4	8	11	15	19	23	26	30	34	38
15 mcg	1.4	3	6	11	17	23	28	34	39	45	51	56
20 mcg	2	4	8	15	23	30	38	45	53	60	68	75

[Microdrops per minute (or mL/hour)]
Contra—↑HR, HTN. ↓dose to 1/10th for patients on MAOIs.
SE—Tachydysrhythmias, VT, VF, HTN, N/V, H/A, ischemia, AMI.

NOTE: Extravasation causes tissue necrosis.

Emerg Meds

Enalaprilat (Vasotec®)   • *ACE Inhibitor/ Antihypertensive*

RX—HTN, Acute MI, CHF: 0.625–1.25 mg IV slowly,
(use lower dose if patient is on diuretics). Repeat in 1 hour if
no response, then 1.25 mg IV every 6 hours.
Contra—Renal impairment, pregnancy, lactation.
SE—H/A, dizziness, fatigue, ↓LOC, dyspnea, ↓BP, angina.

Epinephrine (Adrenalin®)   • *Sympathomimetic*

RX—Allergic Reaction: 0.3–0.5 mg (0.3–0.5 mL 1:1,000) **SQ.**
Peds—0.01 mg/kg (0.01 mL/kg) SQ—maximum: 0.5 mg.

RX—Anaphylaxis: 0.3–0.5 mg (3–5 mL 1:10,000) **IV.**

RX—Asthma: 0.3–0.5 mg (0.3–0.5 mL 1:1,000) **SQ.**

RX—Bradycardia/Hypotension: 2–10 mcg/minute IV.
(mix 1 mg in 250 mL D5W):

Epinephrine Drip

mcg/minute →	2	3	4	5	6	7	8	9	10
microdrops →	30	45	60	75	90	105	120	135	150

> **RX—Cardiac Arrest: 1 mg IV/IO every 3–5 minutes.**
> **Alternative doses for cardiac arrest:**
>   **High Dose: 0.2 mg/kg IVP every 3–5 minutes.**
>   **Endotracheal Dose: 2–2.5 mg every 3–5 minutes.**

Contra—Tachydysrhythmias, severe coronary artery disease.
SE—Tachydysrhythmias, VT, VF angina, HTN, N/V, anxiety.

Etomidate (Amidate®)   • *Sedative/Hypnotic*

RX—Sedation for RSI: 0.3 mg/kg IV slowly.
Contra—Patient <10 years old, pregnancy, do not use with
ketamine, immunosuppression, sepsis, transplant patient.
SE—Apnea, bradycardia, ↓BP, arrhythmias, N/V.

Fentanyl (Sublimaze®) • *Narcotic Analgesic*

RX—Analgesia: 50–100 mcg IM or IV slowly.
Contra—MAOI use, asthma, myasthenia gravis.
SE—↓LOC,↓BP, N/V, bradycardia, apnea.
Peds—1–3 years*: 2–3 mcg/kg IV every 1–4 hours prn;*
        3–12 years*: 1–2 mcg/kg IV every 1–4 hours prn;*
        >12 years*: 0.5–1 mcg/kg IV every 1–4 hours prn.*

Flumazenil (Romazicon®) • *Antidote*

RX—Benzodiazepine: 0.2 mg IV/IO; repeat **0.3 mg IV/IO**,
0.5 mg IV/IO. If patient not responding after total dose of 5
mg, it is not likely a benzodiazepine overdose.

WARNING: Seizure Risk*: Benzodiazepine reversal may
result in seizures in some patients. Cyclic antidepressant
overdose, status epilepticus, ↑ICP, allergy to benzodiazepines.*

SE—Seizure, N/V, agitation, withdrawal. Watch for resedation.
***Peds—0.01 mg/kg IV/IO, up to 0.2 mg single dose, repeat
every minute, as needed. Maximum total dose: 1 mg.***

Furosemide (Lasix®) • *Diuretic*

RX—CHF with Pulmonary Edema, Hypertensive Crisis:
0.5–1 mg/kg IV/IO slowly. Maximum: 2 mg/kg.
Contra—Dehydration, hypokalemia, hepatic coma, anuria.
SE—Hypokalemia, hypotension, dehydration.
Peds—1 mg/kg IV/IO slowly.

Glucagon • *↑Blood Glucose*

RX—Hypoglycemia: 0.5–1 mg (or Unit) IM, SQ, IV.
Give carbohydrate such as prompt meal, orange juice,
D50%, etc., as soon as the patient is alert and can eat.

RX—Beta blocker Calcium-Channel OD: 5–10 mg IV over
1 minute, followed by drip: 1–10 mg/hour.
Peds—0.5–1 mg IV/IO, IM, SQ.

Ibutilide (Corvert®) • *Antiarrhythmic*

RX—Atrial Fibrillation, Atrial Flutter: 1 mg IV slowly over 10 minutes. For patients <60 kg, give 0.01 mg/kg IV slowly over 10 minutes. May repeat in 10 minutes.

Contra—Do not give with class 1a antiarrhythmics such as disopyramide, quinidine, procainamide, or class III drugs such as amiodarone, sotalol. Use caution with drugs that prolong the QT interval: phenothiazines, TCAs, and H_1 receptor antagonists.

SE—PVCs, VT, hypotension, heart block, nausea, H/A, tachycardia, QT prolongation, torsades, HTN.

Inamrinone (Inocor®) • *Inotrope/Vasodilator*

RX—Acute Severe, Refractory CHF: 0.75 mg/kg IV slowly over 2–3 minutes. May repeat after 30 minutes.
Maintenance infusion: 5–10 mcg/kg/minute (mix 300 mg in 240 mL saline = 1 mg/mL).

mcg/kg/ minute	Patient weight in kg									
	20	30	40	50	60	70	80	90	100	110
2 mcg	2.4	3.6	4.8	6	7.2	8.4	9.6	10.8	12	13.2
5 mcg	6	9	12	15	18	21	24	27	30	33
7.5 mcg	9	14	18	23	27	32	36	41	45	50
10 mcg	12	18	24	30	36	42	48	54	60	66
15 mcg	18	28	36	46	54	64	72	82	90	100

Microdrops per minute or mL/hour.

Contra—Hypotension, severe cardiac valve disease. Do not mix with dextrose solutions or furosemide.
SE—Dysrhythmias, ↓BP, N/V, fever, chest pain, myocardial ischemia, hepatotoxicity, thrombocytopenia, burning at infusion site.

Ipratropium .02% (Atrovent®) • *Bronchodilator*

RX—Bronchospasm, COPD, Asthma: 0.5 mg (2.5 mL "fish") nebulized (with albuterol), **repeat x1**.
Contra—Glaucoma, allergy to soy products or peanuts.
SE—Dry mouth, H/A, cough.
Peds—0.25–0.5 mg.

Ketamine (Ketalar®) • *Anesthetic/Analgesic*

RX—Anesthesia: 2 mg/kg IV every 10–20 minutes (or 10 mg/kg IM every 12–25 minutes).
Contra—Hypertensive crisis, allergy.
SE—HTN, respiratory depression, ↑HR, hallucinations, delirium, confusion.

Ketorolac (Toradol®) • *NSAID Analgesic*

RX—Analgesia: 15–30 mg IV or 30–60 mg IM.
Contra—Kidney disease, labor, allergy to ASA or other NSAIDs. Use caution in kidney or liver disease, COPD, asthma, ulcers, bleeding disorders, coumadin use, elderly, diabetes.
SE—Nausea, GI bleeding, edema, HTN.

Labetalol (Normodyne®) • *Antihypertensive*

RX—Severe HTN: (choose either bolus loading dose or infusion loading dose):
Bolus Loading: 20 mg IV over 2 minutes. May double dose every 10 minutes—40 mg, 80 mg, 160 mg, up to 300 mg total dose given.
Infusion Loading Dose: Mix 200 mg (40 mL) in 160 mL of D5W for a concentration of 1 mg/mL. **Start initial infusion at 2 mg/minute and titrate to BP**. May increase up to 6 mg/minute, up to 300 mg total dose infused.

WARNING: Check BP every 5 minutes between doses.

Labetalol Drip (1 mg/mL)			
mg/minute →	2 mg	4 mg	6 mg
microdrops/minute (mL/hour) →	120 gtt	240 gtt	360 gtt

Contra—Asthma, cardiac failure, 2°, 3° block, severe bradycardia, cardiogenic shock, hypotension.
SE—Hypotension, nausea, dizziness, dyspnea.

Lidocaine 2% (Xylocaine®) • Antiarrhythmic

RX—Cardiac Arrest VT/VF: 1–1.5 mg/kg IVP; may repeat with 0.5–0.75 mg/kg IVP every 5–10 minutes. Maximum: 3 mg/kg. **ET dose**: 2–4 mg/kg.

RX—VT with Pulse: 1–1.5 mg/kg IVP; then 0.5–0.75 mg/kg every 5–10 minutes up to 3 mg/kg. Start drip ASAP.

RX—PVCs: 0.5–1.5 mg/kg IV; then 0.5–1.5 mg/kg every 5–10 minutes up to 3 mg/kg. Start drip ASAP.

Drip: 1–4 mg/minute. Mix 1 gm in 250 mL D5W and run at:

Lidocaine Drip (4 mg/mL) →	1 mg	2 mg	3 mg	4 mg
microdrops/minute (mL/hr) →	15 gtt	30 gtt	45 gtt	60 gtt

IM Dose: 300 mg IM (4 mg/kg) of 10% solution.
Contra—2°, 3° block, hypotension, Stokes-Adams Syndrome. Reduce maintenance infusion by 50% if patient. is >70 years old, has liver disease, or is in CHF or shock.
SE—Seizure, slurred speech, altered mental status, ↓HR, N/V, tinnitus.

Lisinopril (Prinivil®) • ACE Inhibitor/Antihypertensive

RX—Hypertension, AMI: 5–10 mg PO.
Contra—Renal impairment, angioedema, pregnancy, hypovolemia.
SE—H/A, dizziness, fatigue, nausea, ↓BP.

Lorazepam (Ativan®) • Anticonvulsant/Sedative

RX—Status Epilepticus: 2–4 mg slowly IV*, or IM.

RX—Anxiety, Sedation: 0.05 mg/kg up to 4 mg IM.
Contra—Acute narrow-angle glaucoma, pregnancy.
SE—Apnea, N/V, drowsiness, restlessness, delirium, ↓BP.

IMPORTANT: Be prepared to ventilate patient.

NOTE: Overdose may be reversed with flumazenil.

Peds—0.05–0.1 mg/kg IV/IO* slowly, or IM. Max: 2 mg/dose.

*For IV/IO use, dilute 1:1 in NS, D5%W, or SW.

Magnesium Sulfate 10% · *Electrolyte*

RX—Cardiac Arrest (Torsades, Hypomagnesemia):
1–2 gm IVP (5–10 gm may be required).

RX—Torsades with a Pulse: 1–2 gm IV over 5–60 minutes
(mix in 50 mL D5W). Start drip of 0.5–1 gm/hour and titrate.

RX—Acute MI: 1–2 gm IV over 5–60 minutes (mix in 50 mL
D5W). Start drip: 0.5–1 gm/hour; run for up to 24 hours.

RX—Seizures 2° Eclampsia: 1–4 gm IV slowly.

Contra—Renal disease, heart block, hypermagnesemia.
SE—Hypotension, asystole, cardiac arrest, respiratory and
CNS depression, flushing, sweating.
Peds—25–50 mg/kg IV/IO over 10–20 minutes. Max: 2 gm.

Meperidine (Demerol®) · *Analgesic*

RX—Analgesia: 50–100 mg IM, SQ or slowly IV.
Contra—Patients receiving MAO inhibitors.
SE—Sedation, apnea, hypotension, ↑ICP, N/V, ↑HR.
Peds—1 mg/kg IV/IO, IM, SQ.

IMPORTANT: Dilute prior to giving IV.

Methylprednisolone (Solu-Medrol®) · *Steroid*

RX—Asthma: 2 mg/kg IV.

RX—Spinal Cord Trauma: 30 mg/kg IV.

Contra—GI Bleed, diabetes, systemic fungal infection.
SE—Euphoria, peptic ulcer, hyperglycemia, hypokalemia.
Peds—Asthma: 2 mg/kg IV/IO, IM.
Peds—Spinal cord injury: 30 mg/kg IV/IO, IM.

Metoprolol (Lopressor®) • *Beta Blocker*

RX—Atrial Fib, Atrial Flutter, PSVT:
2.5–5 mg every 2–5 minutes. Maximum: 15 mg.

RX—Myocardial Infarction:
5 mg IV slowly over 2–5 minutes, repeated every
5 minutes to a total of 15 mg. Then 50 mg orally, every 6
hours x48 hours, thereafter increased to 100 mg twice a day.
Contra—CHF, APE, bronchospasm, bradycardia,
hypotension, cardiomegaly, thyrotoxicosis, Hx asthma.
SE—↓BP, CHF, bronchospasm, ↓HR, chest pain, H/A, N/V.

NOTE: Calcium blockers may potentiate side effects.

Midazolam (Versed®) • *Sedative*

RX—Seizures: 5–15 mg IV slowly, titrate to patient
response. May repeat in 10–15 minutes.

RX—Sedation: 1–2 mg IV over 1–2 minutes, titrated to
effect. May repeat in 2–5 minutes. Maximum total dose: 5 mg.
Contra—Acute narrow angle glaucoma, shock.
SE—Respiratory depression, apnea, ↓BP, ↓HR, H/A, N/V.
May reverse with flumazenil IV.
Peds—Seizures: 0.15 mg/kg IV.
Peds—Sedation: >6 month old child: 0.05–0.1 mg/kg IV
slowly titrated to effect.

Morphine Sulfate • *Analgesic*

RX—Analgesia, Pulmonary Edema: 2–5 mg IV, IM, SQ.
May repeat every 5 minutes up to 10 mg.
Contra—Head injury, exacerbated COPD, depressed
respiratory drive, hypotension, acute abdomen, ↓LOC, labor.

NOTE: Overdose may be reversed with naloxone.

SE—Respiratory depression, ↓BP, ↓LOC, N/V, ↓HR.
Peds—0.1–0.2 mg/kg IV/IO, IM, SQ.

Nalmefene (Revex™)   • *Opioid Antagonist*

RX—Narcotic Overdose: 0.5 mg/70 kg IV, IM, SQ.
(Single IM dose: 1 mg.) Can give second IV dose in 2–5 minutes: **1 mg/70 kg IV.** Maximum total IV dose is 1.5 mg. (Give over 60 seconds in renal failure.)
Contra—Use extreme caution if narcotic dependence is suspected. May try 0.1 mg IV to test for withdrawal symptoms.
SE—Acute withdrawal signs and symptoms, N/V, tachycardia, HTN.

Naloxone (Narcan®)   • *Narcotic Antagonist*

RX—Opiate Overdose; Coma: 0.4–2 mg IV/IO, IM, SQ, ET, IL. Repeat every 2–3 minutes, if needed, up to 10 mg total dose.
Contra—Do not use on a newborn if the mother is addicted to narcotics; may cause withdrawal.
SE—Withdrawal symptoms in the addicted patient, APE, N/V, ↓BP, HTN, seizure.

Nicardipine (Cardene®)   • *Calcium Blocker*

RX—HTN: 5–20 mg/1 hour. Mix 50 mg in 230 mL D5W for 200 mcg/mL. Run at 25–100 mL/hour.

	Nicardipine Drip (200 mcg/mL)			
mg/hour →	**5 mg**	**10 mg**	**15 mg**	**20 mg**
mL/hour (gtt/minute)→	25 mL	50 mL	75 mL	100 mL

Contra—Hypotension, aortic stenosis. Caution with renal failure and hepatic dysfunction.

WARNING: Do not mix with RL.

SE—Edema, hypotension, dizziness, H/A, tachycardia, N/V, facial flushing, vein irritation: change IV site every 12 hours.

Nitrates • *Vasodilators*

RX—ACS, Angina, Hypertension, CHF with APE:
Contra—↓BP, hypovolemia, intracranial bleeding, aortic stenosis, right ventricle infarction, severe bradycardia or tachycardia, recent use of Viagra®, Cialis® or Levitra®, ↑ICP, tamponade.
SE—HA, hypotension, syncope, tachycardia, flushing.

Nitroglycerin tablets (NITROSTAT®)

0.3–0.4 mg SL, may repeat in 3–5 minutes (maximum: 3 doses).

Nitroglycerin paste (NITRO-BID®)

1–2 cm of paste (6–12 mg) **topically.**

Nitroglycerin spray** (NITROLINGUAL®)

1–2 sprays (0.4–0.8 mg) **under the tongue.**

WARNING: Do not shake container.

Nitroglycerin IV (TRIDIL®)

10–20 mcg/minute. Increase by 5–10 mcg/minute every 5 minutes until desired effect. Mix 25 mg in 250 mL D5W (100 mcg/mL) and run at:

Dose in (mcg/min.)	µgtts/minute (or mL/hour)	Dose in (mcg/min.)	µgtts/minute (or mL/hour)
5 mcg	= 3 µgtts/minute	110 mcg	= 66 µgtts/minute
10 mcg	= 6 µgtts/minute	120 mcg	= 72 µgtts/minute
20 mcg	= 12 µgtts/minute	130 mcg	= 78 µgtts/minute
30 mcg	= 18 µgtts/minute	140 mcg	= 84 µgtts/minute
40 mcg	= 24 µgtts/minute	150 mcg	= 90 µgtts/minute
50 mcg	= 30 µgtts/minute	160 mcg	= 96 µgtts/minute
60 mcg	= 36 µgtts/ minute	170 mcg	= 102 µgtts/minute
70 mcg	= 42 µgtts/minute	180 mcg	= 108 µgtts/minute
80 mcg	= 48 µgtts/minute	190 mcg	= 114 µgtts/minute
90 mcg	= 54 µgtts/minute	200 mcg	= 120 µgtts/minute
100 mcg	= 60 µgtts/minute		

NOTE: Use glass IV bottle and non-PVC IV tubing.

Nitrous Oxide (Nitronox®) • *Analgesic*

RX—Analgesia/Sedation: Give mask to patient and allow to self-administer.
Contra—↓LOC, cyanosis, acute abdomen, shock, ↓BP, pneumothorax, chest trauma, patients who need >50% O_2.
SE—Drowsiness, euphoria, apnea, N/V.

NOTE: Ventilate patient area during use.

Ondansetron (Zofran®) • *Antinauseant*

RX—Nausea and Vomiting: 4–8 mg IV slowly, or IM, or 8 mg PO.
Contra—Hypersensitivity to dolasetron, granisetron. May precipitate with bicarb.
SE—H/A, diarrhea, FV, dizziness, pain, seizure, EPS, QT prolongation.
***Peds**—0.1 mg/kg slow IV/IO or IM. Maximum: 4 mg.*

Oxytocin (Pitocin®) • ↑*Uterine Contractions*

RX—Postpartum Hemorrhage: 10 units IM after placenta delivers. Or mix 10–40 units in 1,000 mL balanced salt solution and titrate to control uterine bleeding.
Contra—Rule out multiple fetuses before administration.
SE—HTN, dysrhythmias, N/V, anaphylactic reaction.

Pancuronium *(Pavulon®)* • *Paralytic*

RX—Paralysis to Facilitate Tracheal Intubation:
0.04–0.1 mg/kg IVP (onset 3 minutes; recovery: 30–45 minutes). Maintenance: 0.01 mg/kg every 60 minutes.
Contra—1st trimester pregnancy; use reduced dose in newborns, myasthenia gravis.
SE—Apnea, prolonged paralysis, tachycardia, hypotension, hypertension.

Phenobarbital (Luminal®) • *Anticonvulsant*

RX—Status Epilepticus: 10–20 mg/kg IV slowly, or IM.
Contra—Porphyria, pulmonary or hepatic dysfunction.
SE—Respiratory depression, hypotension, coma, N/V.
Peds—*10–20 mg/kg IV/IO slowly, or IM. May repeat.*

Phenytoin (Dilantin®) • *Anticonvulsant*

RX—Seizures: 10–20 mg/kg IV/IO slowly
(maximum: 50 mg/minute).
Contra—Hypoglycemic seizures (give glucose), ↓HR,
second degree or third degree heart block, impaired hepatic
or renal function, ↓BP, hyperglycemia.
SE—Lethargy, H/A, irritability, restlessness, vertigo,
hypotension, bradycardia.

WARNING: Caustic to veins. Use central line if possible.
Flush line after each dose.

Peds—*15–20 mg/kg over 30 minutes. Maximum: 1 gm.*

Promethazine (Phenergan®) • *Antiemetic/Sedative*

RX—Nausea and Vomiting: 12.5–25 mg IV, IM, or 25 mg PO.

RX—Sedation: 25–50 mg IV, IM, PO.
Contra—<2 years old, allergy to antihistamines and
phenothiazines, lactating females, MAOI use, COPD, HTN,
pregnancy.

WARNING: May cause respiratory depression, severe tissue
injury, gangrene.

SE—Drowsiness, viscous bronchial secretions, urinary
urgency, EPS, confusion, ↑HR, ↓HR.
Peds—Nausea and Vomiting: *0.25–1 mg/kg IV/IO, PO.*
Peds—Sedation: *0.5–1 mg/kg IV/IO.*

Propranolol (Inderal®) • Beta Blocker

RX—VT, VF, Atrial Fib, Atrial Flutter, PSVT, HTN:
RX—Myocardial Salvage for:
• Acute Anterior MI with HTN and Tachycardia
• Large MI <6 hours old
• Refractory cx Pain or Tachycardia 2° excess sympathetic tone
**1–3 mg IV slowly over 2–5 minutes. Repeat dose after
2 minutes to a total of 0.1 mg/kg.** Then 180–320 mg/day
orally in divided doses.
Contra—CHF, APE, bronchospasm, Hx asthma, COPD,
bradycardia, second degree or third degree heart block,
hypotension, cardiogenic shock.
SE—Hypotension, CHF, bronchospasm, bradycardia,
dizziness, N/V.

WARNING: Use of calcium blockers may potentiate side effects.

Reteplase (Retavase®) • Fibrinolytic

**RX—Acute MI (<12 hours old): 10 units IV over 2 minutes.
Repeat dose in 30 minutes.** (Flush with NS before and after.)
Contra—Active internal bleeding. Any within 3 months: stroke,
AV malformation, neoplasm, aneurysm, recent trauma, recent
surgery. Bleeding disorders, LP within 7 days. See *ACLS
section, Stemi Fibrinolytic Protocol* for more contraindications.
SE—Dysrhythmias, bleeding, ↓BP, shock, fever, allergy.

Sodium Bicarbonate 8.4% • Alkalinizer

RX—Cardiac Arrest with Good Ventilation: 1 mEq/kg IV,
(1 mL/kg) followed by 0.5 mEq/kg every 10 minutes.

**RX—Hyperkalemia; OD of: Tricyclic, Phenobarbital,
Diphenhydramine, ASA, Cocaine: 1 mEq/kg IV.**
SE—Metabolic alkalosis, ↓K⁺, fluid overload.

IMPORTANT: Must ventilate patient after administration.

WARNING: Tissue necrosis may occur with extravasation.

Contra—Alkalosis, hypocalcemia, CHF, hypovolemia,
hypernatremia.

Streptokinase (Streptase®) • *Fibrinolytic*

RX—Acute MI (<12 hours old): 1,500,000 units infused over 60 minutes.

RX—Pulmonary Embolism: 250,000 units over 30 minutes. Follow with infusion of 100,000 units/hour.
Contra—Active internal bleeding within 21 days. Surgery or trauma within 14 days. Aortic dissection, severe HTN, bleeding disorders, prolonged CPR with thoracic trauma, lumbar puncture within 7 days, arterial puncture at a noncompressible site. Any within 3 months: stroke, AV malformation, neoplasm, aneurysm, recent trauma, recent surgery. Streptokinase use within past 2 years.
SE—Reperfusion dysrhythmias, bleeding, shock, H/A, hypotension, allergic reaction, intracranial hemorrhage, N/V, fever.

Succinylcholine (Anectine®) • *Paralytic*

RX—Paralysis to Facilitate ET Intubation: 1–2 mg/kg IV/IO (onset: 1 minute; recovery: 4–6 minutes). (IM dose: 3–4 mg/kg, maximum: 150 mg [onset: 2–3 minutes].)
Contra—Acute narrow angle glaucoma, penetrating eye injuries, burns >8 hours, massive crush injury.
SE—Apnea, malignant hyperthermia, dysrhythmias, ↓HR, HTN, ↓BP, cardiac arrest, ↑K⁺, ↑intraocular pressure.
***Peds**—Smaller children: 2 mg/kg; older children and adolescents: 1 mg/kg.*

WARNING: Use caution in children and adolescents. May cause hyperkalemia, arrhythmias, cardiac arrest.

Tenecteplase (TNKase) • *Fibrinolytic*

RX—Acute MI (<12 hours old): 30–50 mg IVP over 5 seconds.
(For bolus: mix 50 mg vial in 10 mL SW [5 mg/mL] and give:)

Patient weight in kg →	50	60	70	80	90	100
Bolus dose in mL →	6 mL	7 mL	8 mL	9 mL	10 mL	10 mL

Contra—Previous hemorrhagic stroke; other CVA within 1 year, intracranial CA, internal bleeding, aortic dissection.

NOTE: See ACLS section, Stemi Fibrinolytic Protocol, for more contraindications.

SE—Intracranial hemorrhage, dysrhythmias, bleeding, ↓BP, shock, CHF.

Thiamine (Vitamin B₁) • *Nutrient*

RX—Co-administration with D50%W in patients suspected of malnutrition or thiamine deficiency (starvation, severe alcoholism): 100 mg slow IV or IM.
Contra—Hypersensitivity.
SE—N/V, hypotension, rash, warm sensation, anaphylaxis.

Vasopressin (Pitressin®) • *Vasopressor*

RX—Cardiac Arrest (VF/VT): 40 Units IVP/IO.
Contra—Renal impairment, migraine, epilepsy, CHF, asthma, CAD, pregnancy, lactation.
SE—IV site pain, stomach cramps, N/V, angina, diarrhea, trembling, eructation, pallor, hives, wheezing, HTN.

Vecuronium (Norcuron®) • *Paralytic*

RX—Paralysis/ET Intubation: 0.1 mg/kg IVP
(onset: 2–3 minutes; recovery: 30–45 minutes).
Maintenance: 0.01–0.05 mg/kg.
Contra—Newborns, neuromuscular disease.
SE—Apnea, weakness, bronchospasm.
Peds—0.1 mg/kg IV/IO.

Verapamil (Isoptin®) • *Antiarrhythmic*

**RX—PSVT, Rapid Atrial Fibrillation, Atrial Flutter:
2.5–5 mg IV slowly over 2–3 minutes**. May repeat with
5–10 mg every 15–30 minutes. Maximum dose: 20 mg.
Contra—Wide-complex tachycardia, heart failure, impaired
ventricular function, hypotension, shock, sick sinus syndrome,
second degree or third degree block, AF with WPW or LGL, IV
beta blocker use, children <1 year old.

NOTE: Hypotension reversed with calcium chloride
500–1,000 mg IV/IO every 5 minutes.

SE—Hypotension, AV block, bradycardia, asystole.
***Peds**—0.1–0.3 mg/kg IV/IO slowly. Maximum: 5 mg/initial
dose. May give second dose in 30 minutes, up to 10 mg.*

Notes

IV fluid rates in drops/minute

Drip Set	10	12	15	20	60*
30 mL/hour	5	6	8	10	30
60 mL/hour	10	12	15	20	60
100 mL/hour	17	20	25	33	100
200 mL/hour	33	40	50	67	200
300 mL/hour	50	60	75	100	300
400 mL/hour	67	80	100	133	400
500 mL/hour	83	100	125	167	500
1,000 mL/hour	167	200	250	333	1,000

*Standard "microdrip" IV tubing has 60 gtt/mL.
A normal "TKO" or "KVO" rate is 30–60 mL/hour.
(Note that with a microdrip IV set, mL/hour = drops/minute).

Notes

Pulse Oximetry

Ranges	Prehospital Care
Normal: 95–99%	
Mild hypoxia: 91–94%	Give oxygen
Moderate hypoxia: 86–90%	Give 100% oxygen
Severe hypoxia: ≤85%	100% oxygen, ventilate

❖ Falsely low SpO_2 readings may be caused by:
  • Cold extremities
  • Hypothermia
  • Hypovolemia
❖ Falsely high SpO_2 readings may be caused by:
  • Anemia
  • Carbon monoxide poisoning
❖ All starting readings must be interpreted in ratio to patient hemoglobin level.

NOTE: If in doubt, give oxygen in spite of a normal SpO_2.

O_2 Tank Capacities

Tank	Capacity	15 Lpm	10 Lpm	6 Lpm	2 Lpm
C	240 L	16 min.	24 min.	40 min.	2 hr.
D	360 L	24 min.	36 min.	1 hr.	3 hr.
E	625 L	41 min.	1:02 hr.	1:44 hr.	5:12 hr.
M	3,000 L	3:20 hr.	5:00 hr.	8:20 hr.	25 hr.
G	5,300 L	5:53 hr.	8:50 hr.	14:43 hr.	44:10 hr.
H	6,900 L	7:40 hr.	11:30 hr.	19:10 hr.	57:30 hr.

Pediatric Cardiac Arrest

Shout for help, activate emergency response, begin CPR, give O_2, attach defibrillator.

VF or Pulseless VT	Asystole/PEA

VF or Pulseless VT

⇩

⚡ Defibrillate 2 J/kg
Continue CPR immediately
(2 minutes of 15:2*)
Obtain IV or IO access

Still VF/VT? ⚡ Shock 4 J/kg
Continue CPR x2 minutes
Epinephrine IV/IO: 0.01 mg/kg
(1:10,000, 0.1 mL/kg)
every 3–5 minutes *OR*:
ET: 0.1 mg/kg (1:1,000, 0.1 mL/kg)
Consider advanced airway
(ET Tube, supraglottic airway)
Ventilate 8–10 breaths/minute
with continuous compressions.
Use waveform capnography:
If $PETCO_2$ <15, improve CPR.

⇩

Still VF/VT? ⚡ Shock ≥4 J/kg
(maximum 10 J/kg or adult dose)
Continue CPR (2 minutes)
Amiodarone 5 mg/kg IV/IO;
may repeat twice.
❖**Identify and Treat Causes**

⇩

Still VF/VT? ⚡ Shock ≥4 J/kg
(maximum 10 J/kg or adult dose)
Continue CPR (2 minutes)
Verify paddle position/contact

⇩

If ROSC (pulse, BP, $PETCO_2$
≥40 mm Hg), provide
post cardiac care.

Asystole/PEA

⇩

Continue CPR immediately
(2 minutes of 15:2*)
Obtain IV or IO access
Epinephrine IV/IO: 0.01 mg/kg
(1:10,000, 0.1 mL/kg)
every 3–5 minutes *OR*:
*ET: 0.1 mg/kg
(1:1,000; 0.1 mL/kg)*
Consider advanced airway
(ET Tube, supraglottic airway)
Ventilate 8–10 breaths/minute
with continuous compressions.
Use waveform capnography:
If $PETCO_2$ <15, improve CPR.

VF/VT?—Start VF/VT
algorithm on left.
Otherwise: CPR (2 minutes);
repeat **Epinephrine** above.

❖**Identify and Treat Causes**
- Hypoxia
- Acidosis
- Hypovolemia
- Toxins
- Hypoglycemia
- Hyper/Hypokalemia
- Hypothermia
- Pulmonary Thrombosis
- Tension Pneumothorax
- Cardiac Tamponade
- Coronary Thrombosis

*After advanced airway,
8–10 breaths/minute.

104

Pediatric Bradycardia
(with a pulse, but symptomatic)

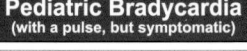

Treat Reversible Causes❖
maintain airway, administer O₂, ventilate as needed,
attach ECG, assess BP, SaO₂,
start IV or IO, 12-lead ECG (but do not delay treatment)

⇩

Severe cardiorespiratory compromise?
(altered mental status, hypotension, shock)

YES	NO

YES

Start CPR if HR <60/minute in spite
of good oxygenation and ventilation
Oxygenate, ventilate

⇩

**Still Bradycardic after 2 minutes
of CPR?** *(If not)*

⇩

Check airway, O₂ source,
ventilation adequacy.
Epinephrine IV/IO: 0.01 mg/kg
(1:10,000, 0.1 mL/kg)
every 3–5 minutes *OR:*
ET: 0.1 mg/kg (1:1,000; 0.1 mL/kg)

⇩

Atropine 0.02 mg/kg IV/IO
(*OR:* ET: 0.04–0.06 mg/kg) for increased
vagal tone or primary AV block
(minimum dose: 0.1 mg; maximum
single dose: 0.5 mg)
[May repeat x1: maximum
total dose: 1 mg]

⇩

Consider Pacing
Treat Reversible Causes❖

⇩

If arrest develops See *Peds Section,*
Pediatric Cardiac Arrest

NO

Support ABCs,
O₂, **Observe,**
Consult with expert

❖Reversible Causes:
• Hypoxia
• Acidosis
• Hypovolemia
• Toxins
• Hypoglycemia
• Hyper/Hypokalemia
• Hypothermia
• Pulmonary
  Thrombosis
• Tension
  Pneumothorax
• Cardiac Tamponade
• Coronary
  Thrombosis

NOTE: Pediatric
bradycardia is often
the result of hypoxia.

Peds

Pediatric Tachycardia
(with poor perfusion)

Treat Reversible Causes❖ (below)
Maintain airway, administer O_2, ventilate as needed,
attach ECG, assess BP, SaO_2, Start IV or IO,
12-lead ECG (but do not delay treatment)

QRS DURATION?

Narrow QRS
≤0.09 seconds

Wide QRS?
>0.09 seconds

Probably Sinus Tach if:

Compatible history?
Normal P waves?
Variable R-R and normal PR?
Infant HR <220/minutes?
Child HR <180/minutes?
⇩
Treat Reversible Causes❖
(below)

Possibly SVT if:

Hx abrupt rate changes?
Absent/abnormal P waves?
HR not variable?
Infant HR ≥220/minute?
Child HR ≥180/minute?
⇩
Consider vagal maneuvers
(do not delay treatment)
⇩
Adenosine 0.1 mg/kg IVP/IO
(6 mg maximum dose)
May repeat with 0.2 mg/kg
(12 mg maximum dose) OR:
⇩
⚡ **Synchronized**
cardioversion
(0.5–1.0 J/kg; may increase
to 2 J/kg if initial dose fails;
sedate if possible, but do
not delay cardioversion)
⇩
Consult expert

❖Identify and Treat Causes
- Hypoxia
- Acidosis
- Hypovolemia
- Toxins
- Hypoglycemia
- Hyper/Hypokalemia
- Hypothermia
- Pulmonary Thrombosis
- Tension Pneumothorax
- Cardiac Tamponade
- Coronary Thrombosis

Go to next page

Wide QRS? >0.09 seconds

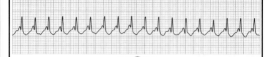

Unstable Patient **(Hypotension, Shock, AMS)**	**Stable Patient**
	Hemodynamically stable?
Possible V-Tach	**Consider Adenosine**
∿ Synchronized Cardioversion	0.1 mg/kg IVP/IO
0.5 J–1.0 J/kg; may increase	(6 mg maximum dose)
to 2 J/kg if initial dose fails	if regular monomorphic QRS
(sedate if possible, but do not	⇩
delay cardioversion)	**Consult expert**
⇩	⇩
Consult with expert	*Either:*
	Amiodarone 5 mg/kg IV over
	20–60 minutes
	OR:
	Procainamide 15 mg/kg IV
	over 30–60 minutes

Pediatric Septic Shock

Recognize altered mental status and poor perfusion.
Give O$_2$, support ventilation, **start IV/IO**, **resuscitate according to PALS**. *Labs:* blood gases (VBG or ABG), lactate, glucose, ionized calcium, cultures, CBC.

⇩

For shock: repeated IV/IO boluses of crystalloid 20 mL/kg (up to 3, 4, or more boluses unless rales, respiratory distress, or hepatomegaly develops)

Additional therapies:
- Correct hypoglycemia and hypocalcemia
- Administer antibiotics immediately
- Consider STAT vasopressor drip (start 2nd IV/IO)   1st hour
- Consider stress-dose hydrocortisone (Draw baseline cortisol; consider ACTH stimulation test. If adrenal insufficiency suspected: give hydrocortisone ~2 mg/kg bolus IV/IO, maximum 100 mg)

⇩

Improved perfusion after IV fluids? ⟶ | **YES** Consider ICU monitoring

NO ◀

Start vasopressor: (titrate to correct hypotension and poor perfusion; consider arterial and central venous access)
Goal: ScvO2 >70%
- **Normotensive?** Start **dopamine** 2–20 mcg/kg/minute.
- **Warm Shock?** (Hypotensive and vasodilated): start **norepinephrine** 0.1–2 mcg/kg/minute. Titrate to BP and systemic perfusion.
- **Cold shock?** (Hypotensive vasoconstricted) start **epinephrine** 0.1–1 mcg/kg/minute. Titrate to BP and systemic perfusion.

YES ◀ ——— ScvO2 >70%? ——— ▶ **NO**

But low BP? *(Warm Shock)*
- Additional fluid boluses
- **Norepinephrine** 0.1–2 mcg/kg/minute. Titrate to BP and systemic perfusion.
- May add **Vasopressin** 0.2–2 milliunits/kg/minute.

go to next page

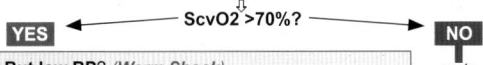

ScvO2 <70%?
Normal BP?

YES ◄─────────────────► **NO**

Normal BP but poor perfusion?
- Transfuse to Hgb >10 g/dL
- Optimize arterial O_2 sat.
- Additional fluid boluses

- *Consider:*
Milrinone 50 mcg/kg loading dose over 10–60 minutes;
drip: 0.25–0.75 mcg/kg/min.
OR:
Nitroprusside
0.3–1 mcg/kg/minute; titrate to response; maximum 8 mcg/kg/minute

---

- *Consider:*
Dobutamine
2–20 mcg/kg/minute

Low BP and poor perfusion?
(Cold Shock)
- Transfuse to Hgb >10 g/dL
- Optimize arterial O_2 sat.
- Additional fluid boluses
- *Consider:*
Epinephrine
0.1–1 mcg/kg/minute
Titrate to BP and perfusion
OR:

Dobutamine
2–20 mcg/kg/minute
+
Norepinephrine
0.1–2 mcg/kg/minute
Titrate to BP and perfusion

Pediatric Medications

Age	Preterm	Term	6 mos	1 yr	3 yrs.	6 yrs.	8 yrs.	10 yrs.	11 yrs.	12 yrs.	14 yrs.
Weight (pounds)	3	7.5	15	22	33	44	55	66	77	88	99
Weight (kilograms)	1.5	3.5	7	10	15	20	25	30	35	40	45
Length (inches)	16"	21"	26"	31"	39"	46"	50"	54"	57"	60"	64"
Length (cm)	41	53	66	79	99	117	127	137	145	152	163
Heart Rate	140	125	120	120	110	100	90	90	85	85	80
Respirations	40–60	40–60	24–36	22–30	20–26	20–24	18–22	18–22	16–22	16–22	14–20
Systolic BP	50–60	60–70	60–120	65–125	100	100	105	110	110	115	115
ET Tube Size (mm)	2.5, 3.0	3.5	3.5	4.0	4.5	5.5	6.0	6.5	6.5	7.0	7.0
Suction catheter size	5–6 Fr	8 Fr	8 Fr	8 Fr	8 Fr	10 Fr	10 Fr	10 Fr	10 Fr	10 Fr	10 Fr
Defibrillation:											
2 J/kg (initial)	3 J	7 J	14 J	20 J	30 J	40 J	50 J	60 J	70 J	80 J	90 J
4 J/kg (repeat)	6 J	14 J	28 J	40 J	60 J	80 J	100 J	120 J	140 J	160 J	180 J
8 J/kg (repeat)	12 J	28 J	56 J	80 J	120 J	160 J	200 J	240 J	280 J	320 J	360 J
10 J/kg (repeat)	15 J	35 J	70 J	100 J	150 J	200 J	250 J	300 J	350 J	360 J	360 J
Cardioversion: 0.5–2 J/kg	1–3 J	2–7 J	4–14 J	5–20 J	8–30 J	10–40 J	13–50 J	15–60 J	18–70 J	20–80 J	23–90 J
Fluid challenge 20 mL/kg IV/IO [Neonates: 10 mL/kg]	15 mL [10 mL/kg]	35 mL [10 mL/kg]	140 mL	200 mL	300 mL	400 mL	500 mL	600 mL	700 mL	800 mL	900 mL

Age Weight	Preterm 1.5 kg	Term 3.5 kg	6 mos 7 kg	1 yr 10 kg	3 yrs. 15 kg	6 yrs. 20 kg	8 yrs. 25 kg	10 yrs. 30 kg	11 yrs. 35 kg	12 yrs. 40 kg	14 yrs. 45 kg
Amiodarone (50 mg/mL) 5 mg/kg IV/IO	0.15 mL	0.35 mL	0.7 mL	1 mL	1.5 mL	2 mL	2.5 mL	3 mL	3.5 mL	4 mL	4.5 mL
Atropine (0.1 mg/mL) 0.02 mg/kg IV/IO	1 mL	1 mL	1.4 mL	2 mL	3 mL	4 mL	5 mL	6 mL	7 mL	8 mL	9 mL
Dextrose (D50%W) 0.5 gm/kg IV/IO [use D25%W for infant]	3 mL [D25%]	7 mL [D25%]	14 mL [D25%]	20 mL [D25%]	15 mL	20 mL	25 mL	30 mL	35 mL	40 mL	45 mL
Diazepam (5 mg/mL) 0.1-0.3 mg/kg slow IV/IO	0.03-0.09	0.07-0.21	0.14-0.42	0.2-0.6	0.3-0.9	0.4-1.2	0.5-1.5	0.6-1.8	0.7-2.1	0.8-2.4	0.9-2.7
Epi 1:10,000 (0.1 mg/mL) 0.01 mg/kg IV/IO	0.15 mL	0.35 mL	0.7 mL	1 mL	1.5 mL	2 mL	2.5 mL	3 mL	3.5 mL	4 mL	4.5 mL
ET Epinephrine 1:1,000 (1 mg/mL) 0.1 mg/kg ET (& 2nd dose IV/IO)	0.15 mL	0.35 mL	0.7 mL	1 mL	1.5 mL	2 mL	2.5 mL	3 mL	3.5 mL	4 mL	4.5 mL
Etomidate (2 mg/mL) 0.3 mg/kg IV/IO	0.2 mL	0.5 mL	1 mL	1.5 mL	2.3 mL	3 mL	3.8 mL	4.5 mL	5.3 mL	6 mL	6.8 mL
Morphine (1 mg/mL) 0.1 mg/kg IV/IO, IM	0.15 mL	0.35 mL	0.7 mL	1 mL	1.5 mL	2 mL	2.5 mL	3 mL	3.5 mL	4 mL	4.5 mL
Naloxone (0.4 mg/mL) 0.1 mg/kg IV/IO, IM, SQ	0.4 mL	0.9 mL	1.8 mL	2.5 mL	3.8 mL	5 mL	5 mL	5 mL	5 mL	5 mL	5 mL
Succinylcholine (20 mg/mL) 1 mg/kg IV/IO [Infant: 2 mg/kg]	0.15 mL [2 mg/kg]	0.35 mL [2 mg/kg]	0.7 mL [2 mg/kg]	1 mL [2 mg/kg]	0.75 mL	1 mL	1.25 mL	1.5 mL	1.75 mL	2 mL	2.3 mL

Pediatric Trauma Score

	+2	+1	-1	Score
Patient Size	>20 kg	10–20 kg	<10 kg	
Airway	Normal	Maintainable without invasive procedures	Not maintainable NEEDS invasive procedures	
CNS	Awake	Obtunded	Comatose	
Systolic BP (or pulse)	>90 (radial)	50–90 (femoral)	<50 mm Hg (no pulse)	
Open wounds	None	Minor	Major or Penetrating	
Skeletal	None	Closed fracture	Open/Multiple Fracture	
			Total =	

>12 = <1% mortality, minimal or no injury
 ≤8 = Critical injury: transport to Pediatric Trauma Center
  4 = Predicts 50% mortality
 <1 = Predicts >98% mortality

Intraosseous Infusion

NOTE: Most medications, blood products, or solutions that can be given IV, can be given IO.

1. **Locate anterior medial (flat) surface of tibia, 2 cm below tibial tuberosity, below growth plate** (other sites: distal anterior femur, medial malleolus, iliac crest).
2. **Prep area with iodine.**
3. Advance IO needle at 90° angle through skin, fascia, and bone with constant pressure and twisting motion. Direct needle slightly away from epiphyseal plate.
4. **A popping sensation will occur (and a lack of resistance) when you have reached the marrow space.**
5. **Attempt to aspirate marrow** (you may or may not get marrow).
6. **Infuse fluids and check for infiltration.** Discontinue if site becomes infiltrated with fluid or medications; apply manual pressure to site followed by a pressure dressing.
7. Secure IO needle, tape in place and attach to IV pump.

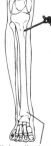

medial malleolus

Pediatric Emergencies—General Assessment

Airway: Look for obstruction, drooling, trauma.
Breathing: Retractions? Respiratory rate? Good air movement?
Circulation: Heart rate? Capillary refill?

WARNING: Bradycardia means hypoxia. Ventilate!

Abbreviations Used on This Page

HX—History, Signs, and Symptoms (black text)

Key Symptoms and Findings (green text)

➕—Prehospital Treatment (blue text with yellow background)

Cautions—Primary Cautions (red text)

Mental Status: Is Child Acting Normally?

HX—Present illness/onset, intake, GI habits. Perform Exam: Fever? Skin color? Other findings?

➕—**Children in shock need aggressive treatment.**
- Ventilate. Reassess the airway, especially during transport.
- Check CBG, consider Naloxone
- IV fluid challenge (20 mL/kg)—repeat if necessary)
- Do not wait for BP to drop—hypotension is a late sign
- Rapid transport to a pediatric intensive care facility

Cautions—Not every seizure with fever is a febrile seizure.
- ✓ Consider meningitis, especially in children <2 years old (check for a rash that does not blanch).
- ✓ Early signs of sepsis are subtle: grunting respirations, temperature instability, hypoglycemia, poor feeding, etc.
- ✓ Consider toxins.

Asthma

HX—Difficulty breathing, shortness of breath, coughing, wheezing, decreased or absent lung sounds, tripod positioning, use of accessory muscles, cyanosis, fever/chills, sputum color, urticaria, skin temp, lethargy. Onset, duration and progression, triggers, response to home treatment. Prior ED admissions. Other possibilities: croup, allergic reaction, foreign body ingestion, etc.

➕—**Improve oxygenation and ventilation**; reduce distress and work of breathing. Monitor: BP, HR, RR, ECG, SpO₂, ETCO₂, serial auscultation of chest. Consider O₂, nebulized bronchodilators: Epinephrine (1:1,000) 0.01 mg/kg (0.01 mL/kg) (maximum dose: 0.3–0.5 mg), administered subcutaneously. For severe asthma: consider Epinephrine (1:10,000) 0.01 mg/kg (0.1 mL/kg) (maximum dose: 0.3 mg), slow IV push every 5 minutes as needed; Solu-Medrol 2 mg/kg IV; Magnesium Sulfate.

Cautions—Remember: "All that wheezes is not asthma."

Croup

HX—Cold or flu that develops into a "barking cough" at night. Relatively slow onset. Low fever.

✚—**Cool, moist air; contact OLMC regarding transport. Consider nebulized epi if age >6 months.**

Cautions—Do not examine the upper airway.

Epiglottitis

HX—Cold or flu that develops into a high fever at night. Drooling, difficulty swallowing, relatively rapid onset. Inspiratory stidor may be present in severe cases.

✚—**Cool, moist air. If airway is completely obstructed, ventilate with BVM and O$_2$.**

Cautions—Do not examine the upper airway. This may cause total airway obstruction.

Notes

Metric Conversions

TEMPERATURE		WEIGHT		OTHER
°F	°C	Lbs	Kg	**Volume**
106	41.1	396	180	1 tsp = 5 mL
105	40.6	374	170	1 tbsp = 15 mL
104	40	352	160	1 fl. oz. = 30 mL
103	39.4	330	150	1 qt = 946 mL
102	38.9	308	140	
101	38.3	286	130	**Length**
100	37.8	264	120	3/8" = 1 cm
99	37.2	242	110	1" = 2.54 cm
98.6	**37**	**220**	**100**	39.4" = 1 meter
98	36.7	**209**	**95**	
97	36.1	**198**	**90**	**Weight**
96	35.6	**187**	**85**	1/150 gr = 0.4 mg
95	35	**176**	**80**	1/100 gr = 0.6 mg
94	34.4	**165**	**75**	1/65 gr = 1 mg
93	33.9	**154**	**70**	1 gr = 65 mg
92	33.3	**143**	**65**	15 gr = 1 gm
91	32.8	**132**	**60**	1 gm = 1,000 mg
90	32.2	**121**	**55**	1 mg = 1,000 mcg
89	31.7	**110**	**50**	1 oz. = 28 gm
88	31.1	99	45	1 lb = 454 gm
87	30.6	88	40	2.2 lbs = 1 kg
86	30	77	35	
85	29.4	66	30	
84	28.9	55	25	**Pressure**
83	28.3	44	20	1 mm Hg =
82	27.8	33	15	1.36 cm H_2O
81	27.2	22	10	
80	26.7	15	7	**"3:00AM Rule"**
75	23.8	11	5	To convert lbs→kg,
70	21.1	7.5	3.5	divide lbs. by 2
65	18.3	5	2.3	and subtract 10%.
32	0	3	1.4	

Common Lab Values

(Adult—blood, plasma, or serum)

NOTE: Normal values may vary, depending on the lab or methods used.

Acetone: 0.3–2 mg%
Alcohol (ETOH): 0 mg%; coma: ≥400–500 mg%
Ammonia: 40–70 mcg%
Amylase: 30–110 U/mL, or 80–180 Somogyi units/100 mL
Aspartate aminotransferase (AST): 5–35 U/L
Bicarbonate (HCO$_3^-$): 23–29 mEq/L
Bilirubin, direct: 0.1–0.4 mg% (total: 0.3–1.1 mg%)
C-reactive protein: <0.8 mg%
Calcium: 4.5–5.5 mEq/L (8.5–11 mg%)
Chloride: 98–109 mEq/L
CO (carbon monoxide): symptoms at ≥10% saturation
CO$_2$ content: 24–30 mEq/L; infants: 20–26 mEq/L
Creatine kinase MB (CK-MB): 0–5 U/L
Creatinine: 0.7–1.4 mg%
Fibrinogen (plasma): 200–400 mg%
Glucose (fasting): 65–110 mg%; diuresis: ≥180 mg%
Hematocrit: Male: 47% (40–50%); Female: 42% (37–47%)
Hemoglobin (Hgb): Male: 14–18 gm%; Female: 12–16 gm%; Child: 12–14 gm%; Newborn: 15–25 gm%
Iron: 75–175 mg% (less in females)
Lactic dehydrogenase (LDH): 132–240 U/L
Lead: <25 mcg%
Lithium: 0.5–1.5 mEq/L (toxicity ≥2 mEq/L)
Magnesium: 1.5–2.5 mEq/L (1.8–3 mg%)
Myoglobin: 10–65 (95 males)
pCO$_2$ (arterial): 35–45 torr; Newborn: 35–40 torr
pH (arterial): 7.35–7.45 (mean: 7.40)
Platelets: 150,000–400,000/cu mm
pO$_2$ (arterial): 75–100 torr (avg–room air at sea level)
Potassium: 3.5–5.0 mEq/L (14–20 mg%)
Protein: total = 6–8.4 gm%
Salicylate: toxicity = ≥30 mg%
Sodium: 136–147 mEq/L (313–334 mg%)
Troponin I: <0.1 mg/mL
Urea nitrogen (BUN): 6–23 mg%
Urine (specific gravity): 1.003–1.030
WBC (leukocytes): 5,000–10,000/cu mm

Labs

Spanish Translations

(In Spanish, "h" is silent; "ll" is pronounced like "y" [yell]; "j" like "h" [ham]; "qu" like "k" [keep]; and "ñ" like "nya" [canyon]. An accented vowel [á, ó, etc.] simply indicates the syllable that must be stressed when pronouncing the word.)

History and Examination

I am a paramedic (firefighter; nurse; doctor).	Soy paramédico (bombero; enfermera/enfermero; médico).
I speak a little Spanish.	Hablo un poco de español.
Is there someone here that speaks English?	¿Alguien habla inglés?
What is your name?	¿Cómo se llama usted?
I don't understand.	No entiendo.
Can you speak more slowly please?	¿Puede hablar más despacio, por favor?
Wake up sir/madam.	Despierte, señor/señora.
Sit up.	Siéntese.
Listen.	Escúcheme.
How are you?	¿Cómo se siente?
Do you have neck or back pain?	¿Le duele el cuello o la espalda?
Were you unconscious?	¿Estuvo inconsciente?
Move your fingers and toes.	Mueva los dedos de las manos y los pies.
What day is today?	¿Qué día es hoy?
Where is this?	¿Dónde estámos?
Where are you?	¿Dónde está usted?
What is your telephone number? ...address?	¿Cuál es su número de teléfono? ...domicilio?
When were you born?	¿Cuándo nació?
Sit here please.	Siéntese aquí, por favor.
Lie down please.	Acuéstese, por favor.

Trouble breathing?	¿Dificultad para respirar?
Weakness?	¿Debilidad?
Where?	¿Dónde?
Show me where it hurts with your hand.	Muéstreme con su mano dónde le duele.
Does the pain increase when you breathe?	¿El dolor aumenta al respirar?
Breathe deeply through your mouth.	Respire profundo por la boca.
Breathe slowly.	Respire lentamente.
Have you been drinking?	¿Ha estado tomando alcohol?
Have you taken any drugs?	¿Ha tomado alguna droga?
Do you have chest pain?	¿Tiene dolor en el pecho?
...heart problems?	...problemas del corazón?
...diabetes?	...diabetes?
...asthma?	...asma?
...allergies?	...alergias?
When were you born?	¿Cuándo nació?
Have you had this pain before?	¿Ha tenido el mismo dolor en otras ocasiones?
How long ago?	¿Hace cúanto tiempo?
Are you sick to your stomach?	¿Tiene náuseas o asco?
Are you pregnant?	¿Está embarazada?
Do you need to vomit?	¿Quiere vomitar?
You will be okay.	Todo saldrá bien.
It is not serious.	No es grave.
It is serious.	Es grave.

Treatment

Please don't move	Por favor, no se mueva.
What's the matter?	¿Qué pasa?
Do you want to go to the hospital?	¿Quieres ir al hospital?
To which hospital?	¿A cuál hospital?
You must go to the hospital.	Tiene que ir al hospital.
We're going to take you to the hospital.	Vamos a llevarte al hospital.
We are going to give you oxygen.	Vamos a darle oxígeno.
We are going to apply a C-collar.	Vamos a ponerle un collarín.
We are going to give you an IV.	Vamos a ponerle un suero.

Miscellaneous

Thank you.	Gracias.	head	la cabeza
Excuse me.	Disculpe.	heart	el corazón
Hello.	Hola.	to help	ayudar
Goodbye.	Adiós.	hip	la cadera
Yes.	Sí.	hypertension	hipertensión/presión alta
No.	No.	leg	la pierna
abdomen	el abdomen	lungs	los pulmones
ankle	el tobillo	meds	medicinas
arm	el brazo	mouth	la boca
back	la espalda	neck	el cuello
bone	el hueso	penis	el pene
cancer	cáncer	stretcher	la camilla
chest	el pecho	stroke	ataque cerebral
drugs	drogas	throat	la garganta
ear	el oído	vagina	la vagina
eye	el ojo	wrist	la muñeca
foot	el pie		
fracture	una fractura		
hand	la mano		

[UPPER CASE = Brand name; lower case = generic name]
(See last pages for abbreviations.)

A

ABELCET (amphotericin B lipid-based): antifungal, Rx: fungal infections

ABILIFY (aripiprazole): antipsychotic, Rx: schizophrenia

Acarbose (PRECOSE): oral hypoglycemic, Rx: diabetes

ACCOLATE (zafirlukast): bronchospasm inhibitor, Rx: asthma

ACCUNEB (albuterol): beta$_2$ agonist bronchodilator, Rx: asthma, COPD

ACCUPRIL (quinapril): ACE inhibitor, Rx: HTN, CHF

ACCURETIC (quinapril/HCTZ): ACE inhibitor/diuretic, Rx: HTN

ACCUTANE (isotretinoin): anti-inflammatory, Rx: severe acne

Acebutolol (SECTRAL): beta blocker, Rx: HTN, angina, dysrhythmias

ACEON (perindopril): ACE inhibitor, Rx: HTN, CAD

Acetaminophen (TYLENOL): non-narcotic analgesic

Acetazolamide (DIAMOX): diuretic/anticonvulsant, Rx: glaucoma, edema in CHF, epilepsy, mountain sickness

Acetylcysteine (MUCOMYST, ACE1ADOTE): mucolytic, antidote, Rx: respiratory diseases, acetaminophen overdose, radiocontrast induced nephropathy

ACIPHEX (rabeprazole): inhibits gastric acid secretion, Rx: ulcers, GERD, Zollinger-Ellison syndrome

ACLOVATE (alclometasone): topical corticosteroid, Rx: rashes, psoriasis

ACTICIN (permethrin): scabicide, Rx: scabies

ACTIFED (triprolidine/pseudoephedrine): antihistamine/decongestant, Rx: allergies, hay fever, cold

ACTIGALL (ursodiol): bile acid, Rx: gallstones

ACTIQ (fentanyl): oral transmucosal narcotic analgesic, Rx: chronic cancer pain

ACTIVELLA (norethindrone and estradiol): oral and transdermal patch, Rx: menopause

ACTONEL (risedronate): reduces bone loss, Rx: osteoporosis, Paget's disease

ACTOS (pioglitazone): oral hypoglycemic, Rx: diabetes

ACULAR (ketorolac): NSAID analgesic, Rx: ocular itching or pain

Acyclovir (ZOVIRAX): antiviral, Rx: herpes, shingles, chicken pox

ADALAT, ADALAT CC (nifedipine): calcium channel blocker, Rx: angina, HTN

ADDERALL (amphetamines): CNS stimulant, Rx: ADHD, narcolepsy

ADIPEX-P (phentermine hydrochloride): adjunct in exogenous obesity, Rx: obesity

ADRENALIN (epinephrine): bronchodilator, vasopressor, Rx: asthma, life-threatening allergic reactions

ADVAIR DISKUS (fluticasone/salmeterol): inhaled steroid/beta$_2$ bronchodilator, Rx: asthma, COPD

ADVICOR (niacin/lovastatin): antihyperlipidemic, Rx: hypercholesterolemia

ADVIL (ibuprofen): NSAID analgesic, Rx: pain

AEROBID, AEROBID M (flunisolide): inhaled steroid, Rx: asthma, bronchitis

AGGRENOX (aspirin/dipyridamole): antiplatelet agents, Rx: to reduce the risk of stroke

AGRYLIN (anagrelide): reduces platelet count, Rx: thrombocythemia, myeloproliferative disorders

ALAMAST (pemirolast): ophthalmic anti-inflammatory, Rx: allergic conjunctivitis

Albendazole (ALBENZA): anthelmintic, Rx: tapeworm

ALBENZA (albendazole): anthelmintic, Rx: tapeworm

Albuterol (PROVENTIL): beta$_2$ agonist bronchodilator, Rx: asthma, COPD

ALDACTAZIDE (HCTZ/spironolactone): diuretics, Rx: HTN, fluid retention

ALDACTONE (spironolactone): potassium-sparing diuretic, Rx: CHF, ESLD, HTN

ALDOMET (methyldopa): centrally acting antihypertensive, Rx: HTN

Alendronate (FOSOMAX): reduces bone loss, Rx: osteoporosis, Paget's disease

ALESSE (levonorgestrel and ethinyl estradiol): prevention of pregnancy, Rx: oral contraceptive

ALEVE (naproxen): NSAID analgesic, Rx: pain

ALLEGRA (fexofenadine): antihistamine, Rx: allergies

Allopurinol (ZYLOPRIM): xanthine oxidase inhibitor, Rx: gout

ALORA (estradiol): estrogen derivative, Rx: menopause

Alosetron (LOTRONEX): antidiarrheal, Rx: irritable bowel

ALPHAGAN P OPTH (brimonidine): alpha adrenergic agonist, Rx: glaucoma, ocular hypertension

Alprazolam (XANAX): benzodiazepine, Rx: anxiety disorders, panic attacks

ALTACE (ramipril): ACE inhibitor, Rx: HTN, CHF post MI

ALUPENT (metaproterenol): beta$_2$ agonist bronchodilator, Rx: asthma, bronchitis, COPD

Amantadine (SYMMETREL): antiviral, antiparkinsonian, Rx: influenza A, Parkinson's disease

AMARYL (glimepiride): oral hypoglycemic, Rx: diabetes mellitus

AMBIEN (zolpidem): sedative, Rx: insomnia

AMBISOME (amphotericin B lipid-based): antifungal, Rx: fungal infections

AMERGE (naratriptan): selective serotonin receptor agonist, Rx: acute migraine headache

AMEVIVE (B 9273, BG 9273, fusion protein-human): Rx: psoriasis

Amikacin (AMIKIN): aminoglycoside antibiotic, Rx: bacterial infections

AMIKIN (amikacin): aminoglycoside antibiotic, Rx: bacterial infections

Amiloride (MIDAMOR): diuretic, Rx: HTN, fluid retention

Amiloride/HCTZ (MODURETIC): diuretics, Rx: HTN, fluid retention

Aminophylline: bronchodilator, Rx: COPD, asthma, bronchitis

Aminosalicylic Acid (PASER): antibacterial, Rx: tuberculosis

Amiodarone (CORDARONE, PACERONE): antiarrhythmic, Rx: dysrhythmias

Amitriptyline: a tricyclic antidepressant, Rx: depression, neuropathic pain

AMITIZA (lubiprostone): intestinal stimulant, Rx: chronic idiopathic constipation

Amlodipine (LOTREL): calcium channel blocker, Rx: HTN, angina

Amoxapine (ASENDIN): tricyclic antidepressant

Amoxicillin (AMOXIL): penicillin class antibiotic

AMOXIL (amoxicillin): penicillin class antibiotic

Amoxicillin/Clavulanate (Augmentin): penicillin class antibiotic

Amphetamine (ADDERALL): stimulant, Rx: ADHD

Amphotericin B (FUNGIZONE): antifungal agent, Rx: fungal infections

Ampicillin: penicillin class antibiotic

Anagrelide (Agrylin): reduces platelet count, Rx: thrombocythemia, myeloprol

ANAFRANIL (clomipramine). tricyclic antidepressant, Rx: obsessive-compulsive disorder

ANALPRAM HC (hydrocortisone/pramoxine): topical steroid/anesthetic, Rx: itching, pain

ANAPROX, ANAPROX DS (naproxen): NSAID analgesic, Rx: arthritis, pain

Anastrozole (ARIMIDEX): estrogen inhibitor, antineoplastic, Rx: breast cancer

ANCOBON (flucytosine): antifungal agent, Rx: fungal infections

ANDRODERM (testosterone): androgen replacement therapy, Rx: hypogonadism

ANTABUSE (disulfiram): alcohol-abuse deterrent, Rx: alcohol abuse

ANTIVERT (meclizine): antiemetic, Rx: motion sickness

ANUSOL HC (hydrocortisone): relief of inflammation, Rx: corticosteroid anti-inflammatory

ANZEMET (dolasetron): antiemetic, Rx: nausea and vomiting caused by chemotherapy, anesthesia, or surgery

APAP (acetaminophen): a non-narcotic analgesic, Rx: mild to moderate pain

APRI (desogestrel and ethinyl): prevention of pregnancy, Rx: contraceptive

AQUAMEPHYTON (vitamin K): Rx: bleeding disorder of newborn

ARALEN (chloroquine): antimalarial agent, Rx: malaria

ARANESP (darbepoetin): erythropoiesis stimulating agent, Rx: anemia

ARAVA (leflunomide): immunomodulator agent, Rx: rheumatoid arthritis

ARICEPT (donepezil): cholinergic enhancer, Rx: dementia associated with Alzheimer's

ARIMIDEX (anastrozole): estrogen inhibitor, Rx: breast cancer

ARISTOCORT (triamcinolone): corticosteroid, Rx: arthritis, severe allergies, asthma

ARIXTRA (fondaparinux): anticoagulant, Rx: treatment and prophylaxis for DVT/PE

ARMOUR THYROID: thyroid hormone, Rx: hypothyroidism

AROMASIN (exemestane): decreases estrogen production, Rx: breast cancer

ARTHROTEC (diclofenac/misoprostol): NSAID analgesic, antiulcer, Rx: arthritis

Ascorbic Acid (vitamin C): prevention of scurvy, Rx: urinary acidification

Aspirin (acetylsalicylic acid, ASA): NSAID analgesic, Rx: pain

ASACOL (mesalamine): anti-inflammatory agent, Rx: colitis

ASTELIN (azelastine): antihistamine, Rx: allergic rhinitis

ASTRAMORPH PF (morphine): narcotic analgesic, Rx: pain

ATACAND (candesartan): ACE inhibitor, Rx: HTN, CHF

ATARAX (hydroxyzine): antihistamine, Rx: itching caused by allergies, motion sickness, alcohol withdrawal

Atenolol (TENORMIN): beta blocker, Rx: HTN, angina, acute MI

Atenolol/Chlorthalidone (TENORETIC): beta blocker/diuretic, Rx: HTN

ATIVAN (lorazepam): benzodiazepine hypnotic, Rx: anxiety

Atovaquone (MEPRON): antiprotozoal, Rx: prophylaxis and treatment for P. carinii pneumonia

ATRIPLA (tenofovir, emtricitabine, efavirenz): antiretrovirals, Rx: HIV/AIDS

ATROVENT (ipratropium): inhaled anticholinergic bronchodilator, Rx: COPD

AUGMENTIN (amoxicillin, clavulanate potassium): penicillin class antibiotic, Rx: bacterial infections

AURALGAN (benzocaine/antipyrine): otic analgesic, Rx: acute otitis media

AVALIDE (irbesartan/hydrochlorothiazide): angiotensin receptor blocker/diuretic, Rx: HTN

AVANDAMET (rosiglitazone/metformin): oral hypoglycemic combination, Rx: diabetes

AVANDIA (rosiglitazone): oral hypoglycemic, Rx: diabetes

AVAPRO (irbesartan): angiotensin receptor blocker, Rx: HTN, diabetic nephropathy

AVELOX (moxifloxacin): fluoroquinolone antibiotic, Rx: bronchitis, pneumonia

AVINZA (morphine ER): narcotic analgesic, Rx: severe pain

AVODART (dutasteride): androgen inhibitor, Rx: benign prostatic hypertrophy

AVONEX (interferon): immunonodulator, Rx: multiple sclerosis

AXERT (almotriptan): selective serotonin receptor agonist, Rx: migraine headaches

AXID (nizatidine): histamine-2 antagonist, inhibits gastric acid secretion, Rx: ulcers

AYGESTIN (norethindrone): hormone, Rx: amenorrhea, endometriosis

126

AZACTAM (aztreonam): monobactam antibiotic, Rx: bacterial infections
Azathioprine (IMURAN): immunosuppressant, Rx: organ transplants, lupus, rheumatoid arthritis
Azelastine (OPTIVAR): antihistamine, Rx: hayfever, allergies
AZILECT (rasagiline): MAO-B inhibitor, slows metabolism of dopamine, Rx: Parkinson's disease
Azithromycin (ZITHROMAX): macrolide antibiotic, Rx: bacterial infection
AZMACORT (triamcinolone): inhaled corticosteroid, Rx: asthma
AZOPT OPTH (brinzolamide): carbonic anhydrase inhibitor, Rx: glaucoma, ocular hypertension
AZT (zidovudine): antiretroviral agent, Rx: HIV
Aztreonam (AZACTAM): monobactam antibiotic, Rx: bacterial infections
AZULFIDINE-EN (sulfasalazine): anti-inflammatory, Rx: ulcerative colitis, arthritis

B

B&O SUP (belladonna/opium): antispasmodic/analgesic, Rx: ureteral spasm pain
Bacitracin: topical antibiotic, Rx: prevention/treatment of superficial infections
Bacitracin/Neomycin/Polymyxin/HC (CORTISPORIN): topical antibiotics/steroid, Rx: skin infection/inflammation
Bacitracin/Polymyxin (POLYSPORIN): topical antibiotic
Baclofen: muscle relaxant, Rx: spasm in MS, spinal cord disease
BACTROBAN (mupirocin): topical antibacterial, Rx: skin infection
Balsalazide (COLAZAL): anti-inflammatory, Rx: ulcerative colitis
BARACLUDE (entecavir): antiretroviral agent, reverse transcriptase inhibitor (nucleoside), Rx: hepatitis B
Beclomethasone (QVAR): inhaled corticosteroid, Rx: asthma
BECONASE AQ (beclomethasone): nasal steroid, Rx: allergies
Belladonna alkaloids with Phenobarbital (DONNATAL): antispasmodic, Rx: irritable bowel
BENADRYL (diphenhydramine): histamine H_1 antagonist, Rx: antihistamine
Benazepril (LOTENSIN): ACE inhibitor, Rx: HTN
Benazepril/HCTZ (LOTENSIN HCT): ACE inhibitor/diuretic, Rx: HTN
BENICAR (olmesartan): angiotensin II receptor antagonist, Rx: HTN

BENTYL (dicyclomine): anticholinergic, Rx: irritable bowel

BENZAMYCIN (erythromycin and benzoyl peroxide): topical skin product, Rx: acne

Benzonatate (TESSALON): antitussive, Rx: cough

Benzoyl Peroxide (PANOXYL): antibacterial, Rx: acne

Benzphetamine (DIDREX): amphetamine, Rx: obesity

Benztropine (COGENTIN): anticholinergic, Rx: Parkinson's disease, extrapyramidal disorders

BETAGAN OPTH (levobunolol): beta blocker, lowers intraocular pressure, Rx: glaucoma

Betamethasone (CELESTONE): corticosteroid anti-inflammatory

BETAPACE (sotalol): antiarrhythmic, Rx: dysrhythmias

BETASERON (interferon): immunomodulator, Rx: Multiple Sclerosis

Betaxolol (KERLONE): beta blocker, Rx: HTN

Bethanechol (URECHOLINE): urinary cholinergic, Rx: urinary retention

BETOPTIC (betaxolol): ophthalmic beta blocker, Rx: glaucoma

BIAXIN (clarithromycin): macrolide antibiotic, Rx: bacterial infections

BICILLIN (penicillin): penicillin antibiotic, Rx: bacterial infections

BIDIL (hydralazine/isosorbide dinitrate): vasodilators, Rx: heart failure

Bisacodyl (DULCOLAX): laxative, Rx: constipation

Bismuth (PEPTO-BISMOL): gastrointestinal, Rx: indigestion, diarrhea

Bisoprolol (Zebeta): beta blocker, Rx: HTN

Bisoprolol/HCTZ (ZIAC): beta blocker/diuretic, Rx: HTN

Bleomycin: antineoplastic, Rx: lymphomas, pleural effusions

BLEPHAMIDE (sulfacetamide/prednisolone): antibiotic/steroid, Rx: eye infection/inflammation

BONIVA (ibandronate): osteoclast inhibitor, Rx: osteoporosis

BRETHINE (terbutaline): beta$_2$ agonist, Rx: COPD, asthma

BREVICON: oral contraceptive

Brimonidine (ALPHAGAN): alpha-2 agonist, Rx: glaucoma, ocular hypertension

Brinzolamide (AZOPT OPHTHALMIC): alpha adrenergic agonist, Rx: glaucoma, ocular hypertension

Bromocriptine (PARLODEL): dopamine agonist, Rx: Parkinson's disease, hyperprolactinemia, acromegaly

Brompheniramine (BROMFED): antihistamine, Rx: allergies

BROVANA (arformoterol): beta$_2$ adenergic agonist, long acting, Rx: COPD

Budesonide (RHINOCORT, PULMICORT): nasal, inhaled corticosteroid, Rx: allergic rhinitis, asthma

Bumetanide (BUMEX): diuretic, Rx: edema, CHF
BUPAP (butalbital, acetaminophen): sedative analgesic,
Rx: tension headache
Buprenorphine: opioid partial agonist-antagonist, Rx: opioid
dependence
Bupropion (WELLBUTRIN, ZYBAN): antidepressant, Rx: depression,
smoking cessation
Buspirone (BUSPAR): antianxiety agent, Rx: anxiety disorders
Busulfan (MYLERAN): anticancer agent, Rx: chronic
myelogenous leukemia
Butalbital/Acetaminophen/Caffeine (FIORICET/ESGIC):
sedative analgesic, Rx: tension headaches
Butalbital/Aspirin/Caffeine (FIORINAL): sedative analgesic,
Rx: tension headache
Butenafine (MENTAX): antifungal, Rx: fungal infections
Butoconazole (MYCELEX-3): antifungal, Rx: vaginal candidiasis
Butorphanol (STADOL): opioid analgesic, Rx: pain
BYETTA (exenatide): enhances insulin secretion, Rx: diabetes (type 2)
BYSTOLIC (nebivolol hydrochloride): beta blocker, Rx: hypertension

C

CADUET (amlodipine/atorvastatin): calcium channel blocker/
antihyperlipidemic
CAFERGOT (ergotamine/caffeine): vasoconstrictors,
Rx: migraine/tension headache
CALAN, CALAN SR (verapamil): calcium channel blocker,
Rx: angina, hypertension, prophylaxis headache, dysrhythmias
CALCIFEROL (ergocalciferol): vitamin D, Rx: hypocalcemia,
hypoparathyroidism, rickets, osteodystrophy
CALCIJEX (calcitriol): vitamin D supplement, Rx: hypocalcemia
in renal disease, hypoparathyroidism, bone disease
Calcipotriene (DOVONEX): vitamin D agonist, Rx: psoriasis
Calcitonin-Salmon (MIACALCIN): bone resorption inhibitor
hormone, Rx: hypercalcemia, Paget's disease, osteoporosis
Calcitriol (CALCIJEX, ROCALTROL): vitamin D supplement,
Rx: hypocalcemia in renal disease, hypoparathyroidism, bone disease
CALDOLOR (ibuprofen): injectable NSAID analgesic, Rx: pain, fever
CAMILA (norethindrone): contraceptive, Rx: amenorrhea,
endometriosis, pregnancy prevention

CAMPRAL (acamprosate): reduces alcohol withdrawal symptoms, Rx: alcohol dependence

CANASA (mesalamine): 5-aminosalicylic acid derivative, Rx: ulcerative colitis

Candesartan Cilexetil (ATACAND): ACE inhibitor, Rx: HTN, CHF

CAPITAL with Codeine (APAP/codeine): narcotic analgesic, Rx: mild to moderate pain

CAPOTEN (captopril): ACE inhibitor, Rx: CHF, HTN, diabetic nephropathy

Capsaicin (ZOSTRIX): topical analgesic, Rx: muscle/joint pain including arthritis

Captopril (CAPOTEN): ACE inhibitor, Rx: HTN, CHF, diabetic nephropathy

CARAFATE (sucralfate): gastrointestinal agent, Rx: duodenal ulcer

Carbamazepine (CARBATROL, TEGRETOL): anticonvulsant, Rx: seizures, trigeminal neuralgia, bipolar disorder

CARBATROL (carbamazepine): anticonvulsant, Rx: seizures, trigeminal neuralgia, bipolar disorder

Carbidopa/Levodopa (SINEMET, PARCOPA): dopamine precursors, Rx: Parkinson's disease

CARDIZEM (diltiazem): antiarrhythmic agent, calcium channel blocker, Rx: angina, hypertension, atrial fibrillation, atrial flutter, paroxysmal supraventricular tachycardia

CARDURA (doxazosin): alpha blocker, Rx: HTN, benign prostatic hypertrophy

CAREFGOT (ergotamine/caffeine): vasoconstrictors, Rx: migraine/tension headache

Carisoprodol (SOMA): muscle relaxant, Rx: musculoskeletal pain

CARTIA XT (diltiazem): antiarrhythmic agent, calcium channel blocker, Rx: angina, hypertension, atrial fibrillation, atrial flutter, paroxysmal supraventricular tachycardia

Carvedilol (COREG): beta and alpha blocker, Rx: angina, heart failure, HTN

CASODEX (bicalutamide): antiandrogen, Rx: prostate cancer

Caspofungin (CANCIDAS): antifungal agent, Rx: fungal infection

CATAPRES, CATAPRES TTS (clonidine): centrally acting alpha agonist, Rx: HTN

CAUDET (amlodipine/atorvastatin): calcium blocker/lipid lowering agent, Rx: HTN and high cholesterol

CECLOR (cefaclor): cephalosporin antibiotic, Rx: bacterial infections

CEDAX (ceftibuten): cephalosporin antibiotic, Rx: bacterial infections

Cefaclor (CECLOR): cephalosporin antibiotic, Rx. bacterial infections
Cefadroxil (DURICEF): cephalosporin antibiotic, Rx: bacterial infections
Cefazolin (ANCEF): cephalosporin antibiotic, Rx: bacterial infections
Cefdinir (OMNICEF): cephalosporin antibiotic, Rx: bacterial infections
Cefepime (MAXIPIME): cephalosporin antibiotic, Rx: bacterial infections
Cefixime (SUPRAX): cephalosporin antibiotic, Rx: bacterial infections
CEFIZOX (ceftizoxime): cephalosporin antibiotic, Rx: bacterial infections
Cefotaxime (CLAFORAN): cephalosporin antibiotic, Rx: bacterial infections
Cefotetan (CEFOTAN): cephalosporin antibiotic, Rx: bacterial infections
Cefoxitin (MEFOXIN): cephalosporin antibiotic, Rx: bacterial infections
Cefpodoxime (VANTIN): cephalosporin antibiotic, Rx: bacterial infections
Cefprozil (CEFZIL): cephalosporin antibiotic, Rx: bacterial infections
Ceftazidime (FORTAZ): cephalosporin antibiotic, Rx: bacterial infections
Ceftibuten (CEDAX): cephalosporin antibiotic, Rx: bacterial infections
CEFTIN (cefuroxime): cephalosporin antibiotic, Rx: bacterial infections
Ceftizoxime (CEFIZOX): cephalosporin antibiotic, Rx: bacterial infections
Ceftriaxone (ROCEPHIN): cephalosporin antibiotic, Rx: bacterial infections
Cefuroxime (CEFTIN): cephalosporin antibiotic, Rx: bacterial infections
CEFZIL (cefprozil): cephalosporin antibiotic, Rx: bacterial infections
CELEBREX (celecoxib): NSAID, Rx: arthritis, acute pain
CELEXA (citalopram): SSRI, Rx: depression
CELLCEPT (mycophenolate): immunosuppressant, Rx: organ transplants
CELONTIN (methsuximide): anticonvulsant, Rx: absence seizure
Cephalexin (KEFLEX): cephalosporin antibiotic, Rx: bacterial infections
CEREBYX (fosphenytoin): anticonvulsant, Rx: epilepsy
Cetirizine (ZYRTEC): antihistamine, Rx: allergic rhinitis, urticaria

Cevimeline (EVOXAC): cholinergic, Rx: dry mouth from Sjogren's syndrome

CHANTIX (varenicline): nicotine receptor stimulator, Rx: smoking cessation

Chloral Hydrate: sedative/hypnotic, Rx: insomnia, pain, alcohol withdrawal

Chlorambucil (LEUKERAN): alkylating agent, Rx: leukemia, lymphomas, Hodgkin's disease

Chlordiazepoxide (LIBRIUM): benzodiazepine, Rx: anxiety, agitation from alcohol withdrawal

Chlorhexidine (PERIDEX): antimicrobial rinse, Rx: gingivitis

Chloroquine (ARALEN): antimalarial, amebicidal agent, Rx: malaria

Chlorothiazide (DIURIL): diuretic, Rx: fluid retention in CHF, renal failure, HTN

Chlorpheniramine (CHLOR-TRIMETON): antihistamine, Rx: colds, allergies

Chlorpromazine (THORAZINE): antipsychotic, Rx: schizophrenia

Chlorthalidone (HYGROTON): diuretic, Rx: fluid retention in CHF, renal failure, HTN

Chlorzoxazone (PARAFON FORTE): skeletal muscle relaxant

Cholestyramine (QUESTRAN): bile acid sequestrant, Rx: antihyperlipidemic

CIALIS (tadalafil): vasodialator, Rx: male erectile dysfunction

Ciclopirox (LOPROX): antifungal, Rx: ringworm, candida

Cidofovir (VISTIDE): antiviral, Rx: cytomegalovirus in AIDS

Cilostazol (PLETAL): vasodilator, platelet inhibitor, Rx: leg cramps

Cimetidine (TAGAMET): histamine-2 blocker, inhibits gastric acid secretion, Rx: ulcers

CIPRO (ciprofloxacin): fluoroquinolone antibiotic, Rx: bacterial infections

CIPRODEX (ciprofloxacin/dexamethasone): antibiotic/steroid, Rx: ear infection

Ciprofloxacin (CIPRO): fluoroquinolone antibiotic, Rx: bacterial infections

Cisplatin (PLATINOL AQ): antineoplastic, Rx: ovarian/testicular/bladder cancer

Citalopram (CELEXA): SSRI, Rx: depression

Cladribine (LEUSTATIN): antineoplastic, Rx: leukemia

CLAFORAN (cefotaxime): cephalosporin antibiotic, Rx: bacterial infections

CLARINEX (desloratadine): antihistamine, Rx: urticaria, allergies

Clarithromycin (BIAXIN): macrolide antibiotic, Rx: bacterial infections

CLEOCIN (clindamycin tropical): antibiotic, Rx: acne, Gardnerella vaginalis

CLEVIPREX (clevidipine): calcium channel blocker, Rx: HTN

CLIMARA (estradiol): transdermal estrogen, Rx: symptoms of menopause

Clindamycin (CLEOCIN): antibiotic, Rx: bacterial infections

CLINORIL (sulindac): NSAID analgesic, Rx: arthritis, acute pain

Clobetasol (TEMOVATE): topical steroid anti-inflammatory, Rx: dermatoses

Clomipramine (ANAFRANIL): tricyclic compound, Rx: obsessive-compulsive disorder

Clonazepam (KLONOPIN): anticonvulsant, Rx: seizures, panic disorders

Clonidine (CATAPRES): centrally acting alpha agonist, Rx: HTN

Clopidogrel (PLAVIX): antiplatelet, Rx: ACS, AMI, stroke

Clorazepate (TRANXENE): benzodiazepine, Rx: anxiety/seizure

Clotrimazole (MYCELEX, LOTRIMIN AF): antifungal, Rx: fungal infection

Clotrimazole/betamethasone (LOTRISONE): topical antifungal/corticosteroid, Rx: fungal infection

Clozapine (CLOZARIL): antipsychotic, Rx: schizophrenia

CLOZARIL (clozapine): antipsychotic, Rx: schizophrenia

Codeine: narcotic analgesic/antitussive

COGENTIN (benztropine): anticholinergic, Rx: Parkinson's disease, extrapyramidal disorders

COGNEX (tacrine): cholinesterase inhibitor, Rx: Alzheimer's disease

COLACE (docusate): stool softener, Rx: constipation

COLAZAL (balsalazide): anti-inflammatory, Rx: ulcerative colitis

Colchicine: anti-inflammatory, Rx: gout

Colesevelam (WELCHOL): bile acid sequestrant, Rx: hyperlipidemia

COLESTID (colestipol): bile acid sequestrant, Rx: hyperlipidemia

Colestipol (COLESTID): bile acid sequestrant, Rx: hyperlipidemia

Colistimethate (COLY-MYCIN M): antibiotic, Rx: pseudomonas infection

COLY-MYCIN M (colistimethane): antibiotic, Rx: pseudomonas infection

COMBIPATCH (estradiol/norethindrone): estrogens, Rx: menopause symptoms

COMBIVENT (albuterol/ipratropium): bronchodilators, Rx: asthma, COPD

COMBIVIR (lamivudine/zidovudine): antiretrovirals, Rx: HIV

COMPAZINE (prochlorperazine): a phenothiazine antiemetic

COMTAN (entacapone): COMT inhibitor, Rx: Parkinson's disease

CONCERTA (methylphenidate): stimulant, Rx: ADHD, narcolepsy

CONDYLOX (podofilox): antimitotic, Rx: anogenital warts

COPAXONE (glatiramer): immunomodulator, Rx: MS

COPEGUS (ribavirin): antiviral, Rx: hepatitis C

CORDARONE (amiodarone): antiarrhythmic, Rx: dysrhythmias

CORDRAN (flurandrenolide): topical steroid anti-inflammatory, Rx: dermatoses

COREG (carvedilol): beta and alpha blocker, Rx: HTN, CHF, angina

CORGARD (nadolol): beta blocker, Rx: HTN, angina

CORTEF (hydrocortisone): steroid anti-inflammatory, Rx: arthritis, colitis, allergies, asthma

CORTIC Ear Drops (chloroxylenol/pramoxine/hydrocortisone): antiseptic/antifungal/steroid anti-inflammatory

CORTIFOAM (hydrocortisone): steroid anti-inflammatory, Rx: proctitis, various skin conditions

CORTISOL (hydrocortisone): steroid anti-inflammatory, Rx: arthritis, allergies, asthma

Cortisone: steroid anti-inflammatory, Rx: various skin conditions, allergies, adrenal insufficiency

CORTISPORIN (neomycin/polymyxin/hydrocortisone): antibiotic/ steroid anti-inflammatory, Rx: ear, eye, and skin infections

CORVERT (ibutilide): antiarrhythmic, Rx: atrial fibrillation, flutter

COSOPT (timolol/dorzolamide): decreases intraocular pressure, Rx: glaucoma

COUMADIN (warfarin): an anticoagulant, Rx: thrombosis prophylaxis

COVERA HS (verapamil): calcium channel blocker, Rx: HTN, angina, dysrhythmias

COZAAR (losartan): angiotensin receptor blocker, Rx: HTN, diabetic nephropathy

CREON, CREON 5, CREON 10, CREON 20 (pancrelipase): pancreatic enzyme replacement

CRESTOR (rosuvastatin): statin, Rx: hyperlipidemia

CRIXIVAN (indinavir): protease inhibitor antiretroviral, Rx: HIV

Cromolyn (INTAL): anti-inflammatory agent, Rx: asthma prophylaxis, allergies

CRYSELLE (ethinyl estradiol and norgestrel): contraceptive, Rx: prevent pregnancy, "morning after pill"

CUBICIN (daptomycin): lipopeptide antibiotic, Rx: bacterial infections

CUTIVATE (fluticasone): topical corticosteroid anti-inflammatory, Rx: dermatoses

Cyanocobalamin (vitamin B-12): Rx: anemia

CYCLESSA (ethinyl estradiol and desogestrel): contraceptive, Rx: prevent pregnancy

Cyclobenzaprine (FLEXERIL): skeletal muscle relaxant

CYCLOCORT TOPICAL (amcinonide): steroid anti-inflammatory, Rx: pruritus, dermatitis

CYCLOMYDRIL (cyclopentolate/phenylephrine): production of mydriasis

Cyclosporine (GENGRAF, NEORAL, SANDIMMUNE): immunosuppressant agent, Rx: organ transplants

CYMBALTA (duloxetine): SSRI, Rx: depression, diabetic neuropathy

Cyproheptadine (PERIACTIN): antihistamine

CYTOMEL (liothyronine): thyroid hormone, Rx: hypothyroidism

CYTOTEC (misoprostol): prevents gastric ulcers from NSAIDs

CYTOVENE (ganciclovir): antiviral, Rx: CMV disease

D

d4T stavudine (ZERIT): antiretroviral, Rx: HIV

DALMANE (flurazepam): benzodiazepine, Rx: insomnia

Danazol: sex hormone, Rx: endometriosis

DANTRIUM (dantrolene): skeletal muscle antispasmodic, Rx: spasm, malignant hyperthermia

Dantrolene (DANTRIUM): skeletal muscle antispasmodic, Rx: spasm, malignant hyperthermia

Dapsone: antibacterial drug, Rx: leprosy, PCP prophylaxis

DARAPRIM (pyrimethamine): antiparasitic, Rx: malaria, toxoplasmosis

DARVOCET-N (propoxyphene/APAP): narcotic analgesic, Rx: mild to moderate pain

DARVON (propoxyphene): narcotic analgesic, Rx: mild to moderate pain

DAYPRO (oxaprozin): NSAID, Rx: arthritis

DDAVP (desmopressin): antidiuretic hormone, Rx: nocturia, diabetes insipidus

DECADRON (dexamethasone): steroid anti-inflammatory, Rx: neoplastic disorders, allergies, GI diseases, endocrine disorders
DECLOMYCIN (demeclocycline): tetracycline antibiotic, Rx: SIADH
Deferoxamine (DESFERAL): iron-chelator, Rx: iron toxicity
Delavirdine (RESCRIPTOR): antiretroviral, Rx: HIV
Deltasone (prednisone): steroid anti-inflammatory
DEMADEX (torsemide): loop diuretic, Rx: HTN, edema in CHF, kidney disease, liver disease
Demeclocycline (DECLOMYCIN): tetracycline antibiotic, Rx: SIADH
DEMEROL (meperidine): opioid analgesic, Rx: moderate to severe pain
DENAVIR (penciclovir): topical antiviral, Rx: herpes, cold sores
DEPACON (divalproex): anticonvulsant, Rx: seizures, bipolar disorder, migraine
DEPAKENE (valproic acid): anticonvulsant, Rx: seizures
DEPAKOTE, DEPAKOTE ER (divalproex): anticonvulsant, antimigraine, Rx: migraine headache, absence seizures
DEPO-MEDROL (methylprednisolone): corticosteroid anti-inflammatory
DEPO-PROVERA (medroxyprogesterone): progesterone, Rx: endometrial or renal cancer
Desipramine (NORPRAMIN): tricyclic antidepressant
Desmopressin (DDAVP): antidiuretic hormone, Rx: nocturia, diabetes insipidus
DESOGEN (etinyl estradiol and desogestrel): contraceptive, Rx: prevent pregnancy
Desonide (DESOWEN): topical corticosteroid, Rx: dermatoses
Desoximetasone (TOPICORT): topical corticosteroid, Rx: dermatoses
DESOXYN (methamphetamine): amphetamine, Rx: ADHD, obesity
DETROL (tolterodine): urinary bladder antispasmodic, Rx: overactive bladder
Dexamethasone (DECADRON): steroid anti-inflammatory, Rx: neoplastic disorders, allergies, GI diseases, endocrine disorders
DEXEDRINE (dextroamphetamine): amphetamine, Rx: ADHD, narcolepsy
Dextroamphetamine (DEXEDRINE): amphetamine, Rx: ADHD, narcolepsy
Dextroamphetamine/Amphetamine (ADDERALL): amphetamine, Rx: ADHD, narcolepsy

136

Dextromethorphan (DELSYM, ROBITUSSIN): non-narcotic antitussive

DEXTROSTAT (dextroamphetamine): stimulant, Rx: ADHD, narcolepsy

DIABETA (glyburide): oral hypoglycemic, Rx: diabetes (type 2 only)

DIAMOX (acetazolamide): diuretic/anticonvulsant, Rx: glaucoma, CHF, epilepsy, mountain sickness

Diazepam (VALIUM): anxiolytic, Rx: anxiety, seizure, panic disorder

DIBENZYLINE (phenoxybenzamine): alpha blocker, Rx: pheochromocytoma

Diclofenac (VOLTAREN): NSAID, analgesic, Rx: arthritis, post-operative ocular inflammation

Dicloxacillin: penicillin antibiotic, Rx: bacterial infections

Dicyclomine (BENTYL): anticholinergic, Rx: irritable bowel syndrome

Didanosine, ddi (VIDEX): antiretroviral, Rx: HIV

DIDREX (benzphetamine): amphetamine, Rx: obesity

DIDRONEL (etidronate): bone metabolism regulator, Rx: Paget's disease, total hip replacement

DIFFERIN (adapalene): topical retinoid, Rx: acne

Diflorasone (PSORCON): topical corticosteroid, Rx: dermatoses

DIFLUCAN (fluconazole): antifungal, Rx: yeast infection

Diflunisal (DOLOBID): NSAID analgesic, Rx: arthritis

DIGITEK (digoxin): cardiac glycoside, Rx: CHF, atrial fibrillation

Digoxin (LANOXIN): cardiac glycoside, Rx: CHF, atrial fibrillation

Dihydroergotamine (D.H.E.): vasoconstrictor, Rx: migraine headache

DILATRATE SR (isosorbide): long-acting nitrate, Rx: angina

DILAUDID (hydromorphone): opioid analgesic, Rx: moderate to severe pain

Diltiazem (CARDIZEM): calcium channel blocker, Rx: angina, HTN, PSVT

Dimenhydrinate (DRAMAMINE): antihistamine, Rx: motion sickness

DIOVAN (valsartan): angiotensin II receptor inhibitor, Rx: HTN, CHF, post MI

DIOVAN HCT (valsartan/HCTZ): angiotensin II receptor inhibitor/ diuretic, Rx: HTN

DIPENTUM (olsalazine): anti-inflammatory agent, Rx: ulcerative colitis

Diphenhydramine (BENADRYL): antihistamine, Rx: allergies

Diphenoxylate/Atropine (LOMOTIL): opioid congener, Rx: diarrhea

DIPROLENE, DIPROLENE AF (betamethasone): topical corticosteroid, Rx: dermatoses

Dipyridamole (PERSANTINE): antiplatelet, Rx: lowers risk of postoperative thromboembolic complications after heart valve replacement

Disopyramide (NORPACE): antiarrhythmic, Rx: ventricular dysrhythmias

Disulfiram (ANTABUSE): alcohol-abuse deterrent, Rx: alcohol abuse

DITROPAN XL (oxybutynin): anticholinergic/antispasmodic, Rx: urinary frequency, incontinence, dysuria

DIURIL (chlorothiazide): diuretic, Rx: fluid retention in CHF, renal failure, HTN

Divalproex (DEPAKOTE): anticonvulsant, Rx: seizures, bipolar disorder, migraines

Docusate (COLACE): stool softener, Rx: constipation

Dolasetron (ANZEMET): antiemetic, Rx: nausea and vomiting

DOLOBID (diflunisal): NSAID analgesic, Rx: arthritis

DOLOPHINE (methadone): Opioid analgesic, Rx: pain, opiate withdrawal symptoms

Donepezil (ARICEPT): cholinergic, Rx: dementia associated with Alzheimer's disease

DONNATAL (phenobarbital/belladonna alkaloids): barbiturate sedative/antispasmodic, Rx: irritable bowel syndrome

DORIBAX (doripenem): carbapenem antibiotic, Rx: bacterial infections

Dornase Alfa (PULMOZYME): lytic enzyme that dissolves infected lung secretions, Rx: cystic fibrosis

Dorzolamide OPTH (TRUSOPT): decreases intraocular pressure, Rx: glaucoma

Dorzolamide/Timolol OPTH (COSOPT): decreases intraocular pressure, Rx: glaucoma

DOVONEX (calcipotriene): vitamin D analog, Rx: psoriasis

Doxazosin (CARDURA): alpha blocker, Rx: HTN, benign prostatic hypertrophy

Doxepin (SINEQUAN): tricyclic antidepressant, Rx: depression, anxiety

DOXIL (doxorubicin): antineoplastic, Rx: AIDS-related tumors

Doxorubicin (DOXIL): antineoplastic, Rx: AIDS-related tumors, cancer, leukemia

Doxycycline (VIBRAMYCIN): tetracycline antibiotic, Rx: bacterial infections

Doxylamine (UNISOM): antihistamine sedative, Rx: insomnia

DRAMAMINE (dimenhydrinate): antihistamine, Rx: motion sickness

Dronabinol (MARINOL): appetite stimulant, Rx: weight loss in cancer, AIDS

DTIC-DOME (dacarbazine): anticancer agent, Rx: melanomas, Hodgkin's disease

DUONEB (ipratropium/albuterol): bronchodilators, Rx: asthma, COPD

DURAGESIC (fentanyl): transdermal opioid analgesic, Rx: chronic pain

DURAMORPH (morphine): opioid analgesic, Rx: moderate to severe pain

DURATUSS AM/PM PACK GP (guaifenesin/pseudoephedrine): decongestant/expectorant, Rx: colds

DYAZIDE (HCTZ/triamterene): diuretics, Rx: HTN

DYNACIN (minocycline): tetracycline antibiotic, Rx: bacterial infections, acne

DYNACIRC CR (isradipine): calcium channel blocker, Rx: HTN

DYRENIUM (triamterene): potassium-sparing diuretic, Rx: edema in CHF/ESLD/nephrotic syndrome

E

Econazole (SPECTAZOLE): topical antifungal, Rx: fungal infections

EDECRIN (ethacrynic acid): diuretic, Rx: CHF, pulmonary edema

EES (erythromycin): macrolide antibiotic, Rx: bacterial infection

Efavirenz (SUSTIVA): antiviral, Rx: HIV-I infection

EFFEXOR, EFFEXOR XR (venlafaxine): antidepressant, Rx: depression, anxiety, panic disorder

ELDEPRYL (selegiline): MAO inhibitor, Rx: Parkinson's disease

ELIDEL (pimecrolimus): topical immunomodulator, Rx: atopic dermatitis

ELIMITE (permethrin): parasiticide, Rx: scabies, lice

ELOCON (mometasone): topical corticosteroid, Rx: dermatoses

ELOXATIN (oxaliplatin): antineoplastic, Rx: colorectal cancer

ELSPAR (asparginase): antineoplastic, Rx: leukemia, sarcoma

EMCYT (estramustine): antineoplastic, Rx: prostate cancer

EMGEL (erythromycin): topical antibiotic, Rx: acne

EMSAM Patch (selegiline): MAO inhibitor, Rx: depression

EMTRIVA (emtricitabine): antiretroviral, Rx: HIV

ENABLEX (darifenacin): anticholinergic, Rx: overactive bladder

Enalapril, Enalaprilat (VASOTEC): ACE inhibitor, Rx: HTN, CHF

Enalapril/HCTZ (VASORETIC): ACE inhibitor/diuretic, Rx: HTN

ENBREL (etanercept): antirheumatic, Rx: rheumatoid arthritis, psoriasis

ENDOCET (oxycodone/acetaminophen): opioid analgesic, Rx: moderate to severe pain

ENJUVIA (estrogen derivative): synthetic hormone, Rx: menopause symptoms

Entacapone (COMTAN): COMT inhibitor, Rx: Parkinson's disease

ENTEREG (alvimopan): GI opioid antagonist, Rx: postoperative ileus

ENTOCORT EC (budesonide): corticosteroid, Rx: Crohn's disease

Ephedrine: bronchodilator, Rx: asthma, COPD

EPIFOAM (hydrocortisone/pramoxine): topical corticosteroidanti-inflammatory/local anesthetic, Rx: dermatoses

EPIPEN (epinephrine): bronchodilator/vasoconstrictor, Rx: allergic reaction

EPIVIR, EPIVIR HBV (lamivudine): antiretroviral, Rx: HIV, hepatitis B

Epoetin Alfa (EPOGEN): increases RBC production, Rx: anemia

EPOGEN (epoetin alfa): increases RBC production, Rx: anemia

EPZICOM (abacavir/lamivudine): antiretroviral, Rx: HIV

EQUETRO (carbamazepine): anticonvulsant, Rx: bipolar disorder

ERBITUX (cetuximab): antineoplastic, Rx: colorectal cancer, cancer of head and neck

Ergocalciferol (CALCIFEROL): vitamin D, Rx: hypocalcemia, hypoparathyroidism, rickets, osteodystrophy

ERRIN (norethindrone): contraceptive, progestin, Rx: amenorrhea, prevent pregnancy

ERYC (erythromycin, systemic): antibiotic, Rx: bacterial infections

ERYGEL (erythromycin): topical antibiotic, Rx: acne

ERYPED (erythromycin): macrolide antibiotic, Rx: bacterial infection

ERY-TAB (erythromycin): antibiotic, Rx: bacterial infection

Erythromycin (EES): an antibiotic, Rx: bacterial infection

ESGIC, ESGIC-PLUS (APAP/caffeine/butalbital): analgesic/muscle relaxant/antianxiety compound, Rx: headache

ESKALITH, ESKALITH CR (lithium): antipsychotic, Rx: bipolar disorder

Estazolam (PROSOM): sedative/hypnotic, Rx: insomnia

ESTRACE (estradiol): estrogen, Rx: symptoms of menopause

ESTRADERM (estradiol): transdermal estrogen, Rx: symptoms of menopause

Estradiol (CLIMARA): estrogen derivative, systemic, Rx: menopause

ESTRATEST (estrogens/methyltestostcrone), Rx: symptoms of menopause

ESTRING (estradiol, topical): estrogen derivative, Rx: menopause

Estropipate (OGEN): estrogens, Rx: symptoms of menopause

ESTROSTEP (ethinyl estradiol and norethindrone): contraceptive, Rx: prevent pregnancy

Ethacrynate (EDECRIN): diuretic, Rx: pulmonary edema, CHF

Ethambutol (MYAMBUTOL): Rx: pulmonary tuberculosis

Ethosuximide (ZARONTIN): anticonvulsant, Rx: absence seizure

Etidronate (DIDRONEL): bone metabolism regulator, Rx: Paget's disease, total hip replacement

Etodolac (LODINE): NSAID analgesic, Rx: arthritis

Etoposide (VEPESID): antineoplastic, Rx: testicular cancer, lung cancer

EULEXIN (flutamide): antiandrogen, Rx: prostate cancer

EVISTA (raloxifene): estrogen modulator, Rx: osteoporosis, breast cancer prevention

EVOXAC (cevimeline): cholinergic, Rx: dry mouth from Sjogren's syndrome

EXELON (rivastigmine): cholinesterase inhibitor, Rx: dementia in Alzheimer's and Parkinson's disease

EXJADE (deferasirox): chelating agent, Rx: iron overload

EXTENDRYL (phenylephrine/methscopolamine/chlorpheniramine): antihistamine/decongestant, Rx: allergies

F

FACTIVE (gemifloxacin): fluoroquinolone antibiotic, Rx: bacterial infections

Famciclovir (FAMVIR): antiviral, Rx: herpes

Famotidine (PEPCID): H-2 blocker, inhibits gastric acid, Rx: ulcers

FAMVIR (famciclovir): antiviral, Rx: herpes

FANAPT (iloperidone): antipsychotic, Rx: schizophrenia

FARESTON (toremifene): antiestrogen, Rx: breast cancer

FAZACLO (clozapine): antipsychotic, Rx: schizophrenia

FELBATOL (felbamate): antiepileptic, Rx: seizures

FELDENE (piroxicam): NSAID analgesic, Rx: arthritis

Felodipine (PLENDIL): calcium channel blocker, Rx: HTN

FEMARA (letrozole): estrogen inhibitor, Rx: breast cancer

FEMHRT (ethinly estradiol and norethindrone): contraceptive, Rx: prevent pregnancy, acne, menopause

Fenofibrate (TRICOR): lipid regulator, Rx: hyperlipidemia

Fenoprofen (NALFON): nonsteroidal anti-inflammatory,
Rx: rheumatoid arthritis, pain

Fentanyl (DURAGESIC): opioid analgesic, Rx: moderate to
severe pain

FERRLECIT (sodium ferric gluconate): hematinic, Rx: iron
deficiency anemia in hemodialysis

Fexofenadine (ALLEGRA): antihistamine, Rx: allergies

FIBERCON (polycarbophil): bulk-producing laxative,
Rx: constipation

Finasteride (PROSCAR, PROPECIA): antiandrogen, Rx: hair
loss, BPH

FIORICET (butalbital/APAP/caffeine): sedative, analgesic,
Rx: tension headache

FIORINAL (butalbital/ASA/caffeine): sedative analgesic,
Rx: tension headache

FLAGYL (metronidazole): antibiotic, Rx: bacterial infections

Flecainide (TAMBOCOR): antiarrhythmic, Rx: PSVT, paroxysmal
atrial fibrillation

FLEXERIL (cyclobenzaprine): skeletal muscle relaxant

FLOLAN (epoprostenol): vasodilator, platelet inhibitor,
Rx: pulmonary hypertension

FLOMAX (tamsulosin): alpha-1 blocker, Rx: BPH

FLONASE (fluticasone): nasal corticosteroid, Rx: allergic rhinitis

FLORINEF (fludrocortisone): mineralocorticoid, Rx: adrenal
insufficiency

FLOVENT (fluticasone): inhaled corticosteroid, Rx: asthma

FLOXIN (ofloxacin): fluoroquinolone antibiotic, Rx: bacterial infections

Fluconazole (DIFLUCAN): antifungal, Rx: yeast infection

Flucytosine (ANCOBON): antifungal, Rx: candida, cryptococcus
infection

FLUDARA (fludarabine): antineoplastic, Rx: lymphocytic leukemia

Fludarabine (FLUDARA): antineoplastic, Rx: lymphocytic leukemia

Fludrocortisone (FLORINEF): mineralocorticoid, Rx: adrenal
insufficiency

FLUMADINE (rimantadine): antiviral, Rx: influenza A virus

Flumazenil (ROMAZICON): antidote, Rx: benzodiazepine
overdose

Flunisolide (AEROBID): inhaled corticosteroid, Rx: asthma

Flunisolide (NASAREL): nasal corticosteroid, Rx: allergic rhinitis

Fluocinolone (SYNALAR): topical corticosteroid, Rx: dermatoses

142

Fluocinonide (LIDEX): topical corticosteroid, Rx: dermatoses
Fluorouracil (ADRUCIL, EFUDEX): antineoplastic, Rx: solar keratosis carcinomas
Fluoxetine (PROZAC): antidepressant, Rx: depression, obsessive-compulsive disorder, bulimia
Fluphenazine: antipsychotic, Rx: schizophrenia
Flurazepam (DALMANE): benzodiazepine, Rx: insomnia
Flurbiprofen (ANSAID): NSAID analgesic, Rx: arthritis
Flutamide (EULEXIN): antiandrogenic, Rx: prostate cancer
Fluticasone (CUTIVATE): topical corticosteroid, Rx: dermatoses
Fluvastatin (LESCOL): statin, Rx: hypercholesterolemia
Fluvoxamine (LUVOX): SSRI, Rx: obsessive-compulsive disorder, anxiety
FOCALIN (dexmethylphenidate): stimulant, Rx: ADHD
Folic Acid: vitamin coenzyme, Rx: megaloblastic anemia
FORADIL (formoterol): long acting beta$_2$ agonist bronchodialator, Rx: asthma, COPD
FORTAMET (metformin): antidiabetic agent, Rx: diabetes
FORTAZ (ceftazidime): cephalosporin antibiotic, Rx: bacterial infections
FOSAMAX (alendronate): reduces bone loss, Rx: osteoporosis, Paget's disease
Foscarnet (FOSCAVIR): antiviral, Rx: cytomegalovirus
FOSCAVIR (foscarnet): antiviral, Rx: cytomegalovirus
Fosinopril (MONOPRIL): ACE inhibitor, Rx: HTN, CHF
Fosphenytoin (CEREBYX): anticonvulsant, Rx: seizures
FOSRENOL (lanthanum): phosphate binder, Rx: hyperphosphatemia in ESRD
FRAGMIN (daltaparin): LMWH, Rx: prophylaxis treatment DVT/PE, ACS
FROVA (frovatriptan): serotonin receptor agonist, Rx: migraine headaches
Furosemide (LASIX): loop diuretic, Rx: CHF, hypertension
FUZEON (enfuvirtide): antiretroviral, Rx: HIV

G

Gabapentin (NEURONTIN): anticonvulsant, Rx: seizures, postherpetic neuralgia
GABITRIL (tiagabine): anticonvulsant, Rx: partial seizures

Galantamine (RAZADYNE): cholinergic enhancer, Rx: Alzheimer's disease

Ganciclovir (CYTOVENE): antiviral, Rx: CMV

Gemfibrozil (LOPID): antihyperlipidemic, Rx: hypertriglyceridemia

GEMZAR (gemcitabine): antineoplastic, Rx: lung, breast, and pancreatic cancer

GENGRAF (cyclosporine): immunosuppressive, Rx: rheumatoid arthritis, psoriasis, prevention of transplant rejection

Gentamicin (GARAMYCIN): aminoglycoside antibiotic, Rx: bacterial infections

GEODON (ziprasidone): antipsychotic, Rx: schizophrenia

Glatiramir Acetate (COPAXONE): biological miscellaneous, multiple sclerosis

GLEEVEC (imatinib): antineoplastic, Rx: leukemia, gastrointestinal cancer

GLIADEL WAFER (carmustine): antineoplastic, Rx: malignant glioma, lymphomas

Glimepiride (AMARYL): oral hypoglycemic, Rx: diabetes (type 2)

Glipizide (GLUCOTROL): oral hypoglycemic, Rx: diabetes (type 2)

Glucagon: hormone, mobilizes glucose, Rx: hypoglycemia

GLUCOPHAGE (metformin): oral hypoglycemic, Rx: diabetes (type 2)

GLUCOTROL (glipizide): oral hypoglycemic, Rx: diabetes (type 2)

GLUCOVANCE (glyburide/metformin): oral hypoglycemic, Rx: diabetes (type 2)

Glyburide (DIABETA, GLYNASE): oral hypoglycemic, Rx: diabetes (type 2)

Glycopyrrolate (ROBINUL): anticholinergic, Rx: peptic ulcers

GLYNASE (glyburide): oral hypoglycemic, Rx: diabetes (type 2)

GLYSET (miglitol): oral hypoglycemic, Rx: diabetes (type 2)

GOLYTELY (polyethylene glycol-electrolyte solution): laxative, Rx: bowel cleansing

Granisetron (KYTRIL): antiemetic, Rx: chemotherapy induced nausea/vomiting

GRIFULVIN V (griseofulvin): antifungal, Rx: ringworm, onychomycosis

Griseofulvin (GRIFULVIN V): antifungal, Rx: ringworm, onychomycosis

Guaifenesin (HUMIBID, MUCINEX): expectorant, Rx: loosen bronchial secretions

Guanfacine (TENEX): antihypertensive, Rx: HTN

GYNAZOLE-1 (butoconazole): antifungal agent, vaginal, Rx: vulvovaginal candidiasis

GYNODIOL (estradiol, systemic): estrogen derivative, Rx: menopause, breast cancer

H

HALCION (triazolam): benzodiazepine hypnotic, Rx: insomnia
HALDOL (haloperidol): antipsychotic, Rx: psychotic disorders
Halobetasol (ULTRAVATE): topical corticosteroid, Rx: dermatoses
Haloperidol (HALDOL): antipsychotic, Rx: psychotic disorders
HCT, HCTZ (hydrochlorothiazide): diuretic, Rx: HTN, water retention
HECTOROL (doxercalciferol): vitamin D supplement, Rx: hypocalcemia in renal disease, hypoparathyroidism
HEXALEN (altretamine): antineoplastic, Rx: ovarian cancer
HUMALOG (insulin lispro): hypoglycemic, Rx: diabetes
HUMIBID (guaifenesin): expectorant, Rx: loosen bronchial secretions
HUMIRA (adalimumab): immunomodulator, Rx: rheumatoid and psoriatic arthritis, ankylosing spondylitis, Crohn's disease
HUMULIN R (regular insulin): hypoglycemic, Rx: diabetes
HYCAMTIN (topotecan): antineoplastic, Rx: lung cancer
HYCODAN (hydrocodone/homatropine): narcotic antitussive
HYCOTUSS (hydrocodone/guaifenesin): narcotic antitussive/ expectorant
Hydralazine (APRESOLINE): vasodilator, Rx: HTN, CHF
Hydrochlorothiazide (HCTZ): thiazide diuretic, Rx: HTN, water retention
Hydrocodone/APAP (NORCO, LORTAB, VICODIN): narcotic analgesic compound, Rx: moderate to severe pain
Hydrocortisone (CORTEF): topical corticosteroid, Rx: dermatoses
HYDRODIURIL (HCTZ): diuretic, Rx: HTN, water retention
Hydromorphone (DILAUDID): opioid analgesic, Rx: moderate to severe pain
Hydroxychloroquine (PLAQUENIL): antimalarial, Rx: malaria, lupus, rheumatoid arthritis
Hydroxyurea (DROXIA, HYDREA): antineoplastic, elastogenic, Rx: melanoma, leukemia, ovarian cancer, sickle cell anemia
Hydroxyzine (ATARAX, VISTARIL): antihistamine, Rx: allergies, anxiety, sedation
Hyoscyamine (LEVSIN): antispasmodic, Rx: lower urinary tract and GI tract spasm/secretions
HYTRIN (terazosin): alpha blocker, Rx: BPH, HTN

HYZAAR (losartan/HCTZ): angiotensin receptor blocker, Rx: HTN

I

Ibuprofen (ADVIL, MOTRIN): NSAID analgesic, Rx: arthritis, mild to moderate pain
Ibutilide (CORVERT): antiarrhythmic, Rx: atrial fibrillation, atrial flutter
Idarubicin (IDAMYCIN): antineoplastic, Rx: AML
Ifosfamide (IFEX): antineoplastic, Rx: testicular cancer
IMDUR (isosorbide mononitrate): vasodilator long acting nitrate, Rx: angina
Imipenem/Cilastatin (PRIMAXIN): carbapenem antibiotic, Rx: bacterial infections
Imipramine (TOFRANIL): tricyclic antidepressant, Rx: depression, bed wetting
IMITREX (sumatriptan): selective serotonin receptor agonist, Rx: migraine headache
IMODIUM (loperamide): slows peristalsis, Rx: diarrhea
IMURAN (azathioprine): immunosuppressant, Rx: organ transplants, lupus, rheumatoid arthritis
Indapamide (LOZOL): diuretic, Rx: HTN, edema in CHF
INDERAL, INDERAL LA (propranolol): beta blocker, Rx: HTN, angina, cardiac dysrhythmias, AMI, migraine headache
INDOCIN, INDOCIN SR (indomethacin): NSAID, Rx: arthritis
Indomethacin (INDOCIN): NSAID analgesic, Rx: arthritis
INFED (iron dextran): Rx: iron deficiency
INFERGEN (interferon alfacon-1): antiviral, Rx: hepatitis C
Infliximab (REMICADE): neutralizes tumor necrosis factor, Rx: Crohn's disease
INH (isoniazid): antibiotic, Rx: tuberculosis
INSPRA (eplerenone): aldosterone blocker, Rx: HTN, CHF
INTAL (cromolyn): anti-inflammatory, Rx: asthma
INTELENCE (etravirine): antiretroviral, Rx: HIV
INTRON A (interferon alpha-2b): interferon, Rx: chronic hepatitis B/C, leukemia, lymphoma
INVEGA (paliperidone): antipsychotic, Rx: schizophrenia
INVIRASE (saquinavir): protease inhibitor antiretroviral, Rx: HIV
Irinotecan (CAMPTOSAR): antineoplastic, Rx: colon and rectal cancer
IONAMIN (phentermine): anorexiant stimulant, Rx: obesity
Ipecac: detoxification agent, Rx: overdose/poisoning

Ipratropium (ATROVENT): bronchodilator, Rx: COPD
ISENTRESS (raltegravir): antiretroviral, Rx: HIV
ISMO (isosorbide mononitrate): vasodilator, Rx: angina
Isoniazid: antibiotic, Rx: tuberculosis
Isoproterenol: beta bronchodilator, Rx: asthma, COPD
ISOPTIN SR (verapamil): calcium channel blocker, Rx: angina, HTN, PSVT prophylaxis, headache
ISOPTO CARPINE OPTH (pilocarpine): cholinergic miotic, Rx: glaucoma
Isosorbide dinitrate (ISORDIL): nitrate vasodilator, Rx: angina
Isosorbide mononitrate (IMDUR, ISMO, MONOKET): long-acting nitrate, Rx: angina
Isradipine (DYNACIRC): calcium channel blocker, Rx: HTN
Itraconazole (SPORANOX): antifungal, Rx: fungal infections

J

JANUMET (sitagliptin/metformin): oral hypoglycemics, Rx: diabetes (type 2)
JANUVIA (sitagliptin): oral hypoglycemic, Rx: diabetes (type 2)
JOLIVETTE (norethindrone): contraceptive, progestin, Rx: amenorrhea, prevent pregnancy, endometriosis
JUNEL (ethinyl estradiol and norethindrone): contraceptive, Rx: prevent pregnancy, acne, menopause

K

KADIAN (morphine ER): opioid analgesic, Rx: severe pain
KALETRA (lopinavir/ritonavir): antiretrovirals, Rx: HIV
KAOPECTATE (bismuth): gastrointestinal, Rx: indigestion, diarrhea
Kanamycin (KANTREX): aminoglycoside antibiotic, Rx: bacterial infection
KAPIDEX (dexlansoprazole): proton pump inhibitor, Rx: GERD, erosive esophagitis
KAYEXALATE (sodium polystyrene sulfonate): antidote, Rx: hyperkalemia
K-DUR (potassium): electrolyte, Rx: hypokalemia
KEFLEX (cephalexin): cephalosporin antibiotic, Rx: bacterial infections
KEPPRA (levatiracetam): anticonvulsant, Rx: seizures

KERLONE (betaxolol): beta-1 blocker, Rx: HTN
KETEK (telithromycin): ketolide antibiotic, Rx: community acquired PNA
Ketoconazole (NIZORAL): antifungal agent, Rx: fungal infections
Ketoprofen: NSAID analgesic, Rx: arthritis
Ketorolac (TORADOL): NSAID analgesic, Rx: acute pain
Ketotifen OPTH (ZADITOR): antihistamine, anti-inflammatory, Rx: allergic conjunctivitis
KINERET (anakinra): antirheumatic, disease modifying, Rx: rheumatoid arthritis
KLONOPIN (clonazepam): benzodiazepine hypnotic, Rx: seizures, panic disorder
KLOR-CON (potassium): electrolyte, Rx: hypokalemia
KOGENATE (antihemophilic Factor VIII): Rx: hemophilia
KONSYL (psyllium): bulk-forming laxative, Rx: constipation
KRISTALOSE (lactulose): ammonium detoxicant, laxative, Rx: constipation
KUTRASE (pancreatin): pancreatic enzymes replacement in CF, chronic pancreatitis
KWELL (lindane): parasiticide, Rx: lice, scabies
KYTRIL (granisetron): antiemetic, Rx: chemotherapy induced nausea/vomiting

L

Labetalol (TRANDATE): beta blocker, Rx: HTN
LAC-HYDRIN (ammonium lactate): emollient, Rx: dry, itchy skin
LACRI-LUBE OPTH (white petrolatum/mineral oil): Rx: ophthalmic lubrication
LACRISERT (hydroxypropyl): opthalmic lubricant, Rx: dry eyes
Lactulose (CEPHULAC): hyperosmotic laxative, Rx: constipation, encephalopathy
LAMICTAL (lamotrigine): anticonvulsant, Rx: seizures, bipolar disorder
LAMISIL (terbinafine): antifungal, Rx: fungal infections
Lamivudine (EPIVIR): antiviral, Rx: HIV
Lamotrigine (LAMICTAL): anticonvulsant, Rx: seizures, bipolar disorder
LANOXIN (digoxin): cardiac glycoside, Rx: CHF, atrial fibrillation
Lansoprazole (PREVACID): gastric acid pump inhibitor, Rx: ulcers, GERD

LANTUS (insulin glargine): hypoglycemic, Rx: diabetes
LARIAM (mefloquine): antimalarial agent
LASIX (furosemide): loop diuretic, Rx: HTN, CHF
Leflunomide (ARAVA): immunomodulator, anti-inflammatory, Rx: rheumatoid arthritis
LESCOL (fluvastatin): statin, Rx: hypercholesterolemia
LESSINA (ethinyl estradiol and levonorgestrel): contraceptive, Rx: prevent pregnancy
LEUKERAN (chlorambucil): antineoplastic, Rx: leukemia, lymphoma, Hodgkin's disease
Leucovorin: vitamin, Rx: methotrexate toxicity, megaloblastic anemia
Leuprolide (LUPRON): hormone, Rx: endometriosis, advanced prostate cancer
Levalbuterol (XOPENEX): inhaled beta$_2$ bronchodilator, Rx: COPD, asthma
Levamisole (ERGAMISOLE): immunostimulant, Rx: colon cancer
LEVAQUIN (levofloxacin): antibotic, Rx: pneumonia, COPD, UTI
Levatiracetam (KEPPRA): anticonvulsant, Rx: seizures
LEVATOL (penbutolol): beta blocker, Rx: hypertension
LEVBID (hyoscyamine): anticholinergic agent, Rx: peptic ulcer, colic, GI disorders
LEVEMIR (insulin detemir): hypoglycemic, Rx: diabetes
LEVITRA (vardenafil): vasodilator, Rx: erectile dysfunction
LEVLEN (ethinyl estradiol and levonorgestrel): contraceptive, Rx: prevent pregnancy
LEVLIN (ethinyl estradiol/levonorgestrel): oral contraceptive
Levobunolol OPTH (BETAGAN): beta blocker, Rx: glaucoma
Levodopa/carbidopa (SINEMET): dopamine precursor, Rx: Parkinson's disease
Levofloxacin (LEVAQUIN): fluoroquinolone antibiotic, Rx: bacterial infections
LEVORA (levonorgestrel/estradiol): oral contraceptive
LEVOTHROID (levothyroxine): thyroid hormone, Rx: hypothyroidism
Levothyroxine (LEVOTHROID, LEVOXYL, SYNTHROID): thyroid hormone, Rx: hypothyroidism
LEVOXYL (levothyroxine): thyroid hormone, Rx: hypothyroidism
LEVSIN, LEVSINEX (hyoscyamine): antispasmodic, Rx: lower urinary tract and GI tract spasm/secretions
LEXAPRO (escitalopram): SSRI antidepressant, Rx: depression, anxiety disorder
LEXIVA (fosamprenavir): antiretroviral, Rx: HIV

LIBRIUM (chlordiazepoxide): benzodiazepine, Rx: anxiety, alcohol withdrawal

LIDEX (fluocinonide): topical corticosteroid, Rx: dermatoses

LIDODERM (lidocaine) topical local anesthetic, Rx: postherpetic neuralgia

Lindane (KWELL): parasiticide, Rx: scabies, lice

Liothyronine (CYTOMEL): thyroid hormone, Rx: hypothyroidism

Liotrix (THYROLAR): thyroid hormone, Rx: hypothyroidism

LIPITOR (atorvastatin): statin, Rx: hypercholesterolemia, CHD

LIPRAM UL (pancrelipase): pancreatic enzymes replacement, Rx: chronic pancreatitis, cystic fibrosis

Lisinopril (PRINIVIL, ZESTRIL): ACE inhibitor, Rx: HTN, CHF, AMI

Lisinopril/HCTZ (ZESTORETIC): ACE inhibitor, Rx: HTN, CHF, AMI

Lithium (LITHOBID): antipsychotic, Rx: bipolar disorder

LITHOBID (lithium): antipsychotic, Rx: bipolar disorder

LOCOID (hydrocortisone): topical corticosteroid, Rx: dermatoses, seborrheic dermatitis

LODRANE 12D (brompheniramine/pseudoephedrine): antihistamine/decongestant, Rx: allergies, common cold

LOESTRIN (ethinyl estradiol/norethindrone): oral contraceptive

LOMOTIL (diphenoxylate/atropine): opioid congener, Rx: diarrhea

LONOX (diphenoxylate/atropine): opioid congener, Rx: diarrhea

LO/OVRAL (ethinyl estradiol/norgestrel): oral contraceptive

Loperamide (IMODIUM): slows peristalsis, Rx: diarrhea

LOPID (gemfibrozil): antihyperllipidemic, Rx: hypertriglyceridemia

Lopinavir (KALETRA): antiviral, Rx: HIV, AIDS

LOPRESSOR (metoprolol): beta-1 blocker, Rx: hypertension

LOPROX (ciclopirox): antifungal, Rx: ringworm, candida

Loratadine (CLARITIN): antihistamine, Rx: allergies

Lorazepam (ATIVAN): benzodiazepine hypnotic, Rx: anxiety, status epilepticus

LORCET 10/650, LORCET HD, LORCET PLUS (hydrocodone/APAP): opioid analgesic compound, Rx: mild to moderate pain

LORTAB (hydrocodone/APAP): narcotic analgesic

Losartan (COZAAR): angiotensin receptor blocker, Rx: HTN, diabetic nephropathy

LOTENSIN (benazepril): ACE inhibitor, Rx: HTN, CHF

LOTENSIN HCT (benazepril/HCTZ): ACE inhibitor/diuretic, Rx: HTN

LOTREL (amlodipine/benazepril): calcium channel blocker/ACE inhibitor, Rx: HTN

LOTRIMIN (clotrimazole): topical antifungal agent, Rx: fungal infections

LOTRISONE (clotrimazole/betamethasone): topical antifungal/corticosteroid, Rx: fungal infections

LOTRONEX (alosetron): antidiarrheal, Rx: irritable bowel syndrome

Lovastatin (MEVACOR): statin, Rx: hypercholesterolemia, CHD

LOVENOX (enoxaparin): LMWH, Rx: prophylaxis/tx DVT/PE, ACS

LOW-OGESTREL (ethinyl estradiol and norgestrel): contraceptive, Rx: prevent pregnancy, "morning after pill"

Loxapine (LOXITANE): antipsychotic, Rx: schizophrenia

LOXITANE (loxapine): antipsychotic, Rx: schizophrenia

LOZOL (indapamide): diuretic, Rx: HTN, edema in CHF

LUCENTIS (ranibizumab): blood vessel growth inhibitor, Rx: macular degeneration

LUMIGAN OPTH (bimatoprost): lowers intraocular pressure, Rx: glaucoma

LUNESTA (eszopiclone): sedative, Rx: insomnia

LUPRON DEPOT (leuprolide): hormone, Rx: endometriosis, prostrate cancer

LUVOX (fluvoxamine): SSRI antidepressant, Rx: obsessive-compulsive disorder, anxiety

LYRICA (pregabalin): anticonvulsant, Rx: partial seizures, neuropathic pain

M

MAFENIDE (sulfamylon): topical antimicrobial, Rx: burn wounds

MACROBID (nitrofurantoin): nitrofuran antibiotic, Rx: UTI

MACRODANTIN (nitrofurantoin): nitrofuran antibiotic, Rx: UTI

MALARONE (atovaquone/proguanil): antimalarial agents, Rx: malaria prevention/treatment

Malathion (OVIDE): organophosphate insecticide, Rx: head lice

Mannitol (OSMITROL): osmotic diuretic, Rx: cerebral edema, IOP

Maprotiline (LUDIOMIL): tetracyclic antidepressant, Rx: depression, bipolar disorder, anxiety

MARINOL (dronabinol): appetite stimulant, Rx: weight loss in cancer, AIDS

MAVIK (trandolapril): ACE inhibitor, Rx: HTN, CHF post MI

MAXAIR (pirbuterol): inhaled beta$_2$ stimulant, Rx: asthma, COPD

MAXALT (rizatriptan): selective serotonin receptor agonist, Rx: migraine headaches

MAXIDEX OPTH (dexamethasone): corticosteroid, Rx: corneal injury, allergic conjunctivitis

MAXITROL OPTH (neomycin/polymyxin/dexamethasone): antibiotics/steroid, Rx: eye infection/inflammation

MAXZIDE (triamterene/HCTZ): diuretics, Rx: HTN, water retention

MEBARAL (mephobarbital): barbiturate sedative, Rx: epilepsy, anxiety

Mebendazole (VERMOX): anthelmintic, Rx: intestinal worms

Meclizine (ANTIVERT): antinauseant, Rx: motion sickness

Meclofenamate: NSAID analgesic, Rx: arthritis, acute pain

MEDROL (methylprednisolone): glucocorticoid, Rx: adrenal insufficiency, allergies, RA

Medroxyprogesterone (PROVERA): progestin hormone, Rx: endometriosis, amenorrhea, uterine bleeding, contraception

MEFOXIN (cefoxitin): cephalosporin antibiotic, Rx: bacterial infections

Mefloquine (LARIAM): antimalarial, Rx: prevention and treatment of malaria

Megestrol (MEGACE): progestin, appetite stimulant, Rx: anorexia with AIDS, antineoplastic, Rx: breast cancer, endometrial cancer

Meloxicam (MOBIC): NSAID analgesic, Rx: arthritis

MENTAX (butenafine): topical antifungal, Rx: ringworm, athlete's foot

Meperidine (DEMEROL): opioid analgesic, Rx: moderate to severe pain

MEPHYTON (vitamin K-1): Rx: coagulation disorders

Meprobamate (MILTOWN): antianxiety agent, Rx: anxiety disorders

MEPRON (atovaquone): antiprotozoal, Rx: prophylaxis and treatment for pneumocystic carinii pneumonia in AIDS

Mercaptopurine (PURINETHOL): antineoplastic, Rx: leukemia

MERIDIA (sibutramine): stimulant, Rx: obesity

MERREM (meropenem): carbapenem antibiotic, Rx: bacterial infections

Mesalamine (ASACOL, PENTASA): anti-inflammatory agent, Rx: ulcerative colitis

MESTINON (pyridostigmine): anticholinesterase, Rx: myasthenia gravis

METADATE CD, ER (methylphenidate): stimulant, Rx: ADHD, narcolepsy

METAGLIP (glipizide/metformin): oral hypoglycemics, Rx: diabetes (type 2)

Metaproterenol (ALUPENT): beta$_2$ agonist bronchodilator, Rx: COPD, asthma

Metformin (GLUCOPHAGE): oral hypoglycemic, Rx: diabetes (type 2)

Methadone (DOLOPHINE): opioid analgesic, Rx: moderate to severe pain, opiate withdrawal

METHADOSE (methadone): analgesic, opioid, Rx: detoxification of opioid addiction

Methenamine (URISED, UREX): antibiotic, Rx: UTI prophylaxis

METHERGINE (methylergonovine): increases uterine contractions, Rx: uterine contraction/bleeding

Methimazole (TAPAZOLE): Rx: antithyroid; Rx: hyperthyroidism

Methocarbamol (ROBAXIN): skeletal muscle relaxant

Methotrexate: antineoplastic, Rx: psoriasis, cancer, rheumatoid arthritis

Methsuximide (CELONTIN): anticonvulsant, Rx: absence seizure

Methyldopa (ALDOMET): centrally acting antihypertensive, Rx: HTN

Methylphenidate (RITALIN): stimulant, Rx: ADHD, narcolepsy

Methylprednisolone (MEDROL): glucocorticoid, Rx: adrenal insufficiency, allergies, RA

Metoclopramide (REGLAN): improves gastric emptying, Rx: heartburn, diabetic gastroparesis

Metolazone (ZAROXOLYN): thiazide diuretic, Rx: HTN, fluid retention

Metoprolol (LOPRESSOR, TOPROL-XL): beta-1 blocker, Rx: HTN, angina, dysrhythmias

Metronidazole (FLAGYL): antibiotic, Rx: bacterial infections

MEVACOR (lovastatin): statin, Rx: hypercholesterolemia, CHD

Mexiletine (MEXITIL): antiarrhythmic, Rx: ventricular dysrhythmias

MEXITIL (mexiletine): antiarrhythmic, Rx: ventricular dysrhythmias

MIACALCIN (calcitonin-salmon): bone resorption inhibitor hormone, Rx: hypercalcemia, Paget's disease, osteoporosis

MICARDIS (telmisartan): angiotensin II receptor antagonist, Rx: HTN

Miconazole (MONISTAT): antifungal, Rx: candidiasis

MICRO-K (potassium): electrolyte, Rx: hypokalemia

MICROZIDE (HCTZ): thiazide diuretic, Rx: HTN, water retention

MIDAMOR (amiloride): potassium-sparing diuretic, Rx: HTN, CHF

Midazolam: benzodiazepine hypnotic, Rx: anxiety before surgery

Midodrine (PROAMATINE): vasopressor, Rx: orthostatic hypotension

MIDRIN (isometheptene, dichloralphenazone, APAP): vasoconstrictor/sedative/analgesic, Rx: migraines

MINIPRESS (prazosin): alpha-1 blocker, Rx: hypertension

MINITRAN (transdermal nitroglycerin): nitrate, Rx: angina
MINOCIN (minocycline): tetracycline antibiotic, Rx: bacterial infections, acne
Minocycline (MINOCIN): tetracycline antibiotic, Rx: bacterial infections, acne
Minoxidil: vasodilator, Rx: severe HTN
MIRALAX (polyethylene glycol): osmotic laxative, Rx: constipation
MIRAPEX (pramipexole): dopamine agonist, Rx: Parkinson's disease, restless legs syndrome
MIRCERA (methoxypolyethyleneglycol-epoetin): increases RBC production, Rx: anemia in chronic renal failure
Mirtazapine (REMERON): antidepressant, Rx: depression
Misoprostol (CYTOTEC): antiulcer, Rx: NSAID-induced gastric ulcers
MOBIC (meloxicam): NSAID analgesic, Rx: athritis
Modafinil (PROVIGIL): wakefulness-promoting agent, Rx: narcolepsy, daytime sleepiness
MODURETIC (amiloride/HCTZ): diuretics, Rx: HTN, fluid retention
Moexipril (UNIVASC): ACE inhibitor, Rx: HTN
Mometasone (ELOCON): topical corticosteroid, Rx: dermatoses
MONOCAL (fluoride, calcium): mineral supplement
MONOKET (isosorbide mononitrate): long acting nitrate, Rx: angina
MONOPRIL (fosinopril): ACE inhibitor, Rx: HTN, CHF
MONUROL (fosfomycin): antibiotic, Rx: UTI
Morphine sulfate (MS CONTIN): opioid analgesic, Rx: moderate to severe pain
MOTOFEN (difenoxin/atropine): decreases intestinal motility, Rx: diarrhea
Moxifloxacin (AVELOX): fluoroquinolone antibiotic, Rx: bacterial infections
MS CONTIN (morphine ER): narcotic analgesic, Rx: moderate to severe pain
MUCINEX (guaifenesin): expectorant, Rx: loosen bronchial secretions
Mupirocin (BACTROBAN): topical antibiotic, Rx: topical infections
MYCELEX 3 (butoconazole): vaginal antifungal, Rx: yeast infection
MYCOBUTIN (rifabutin): antibiotic, Rx: mycobacterium avium complex in HIV
Mycophenolate (CELLCEPT): immunosuppressant, Rx: organ transplants
MYCOSTATIN (nystatin): antifungal, Rx: candidiasis
MYLERAN (busulfan): alkylating agent, Rx: leukemia

MYSOLINE (primidone): anticonvulsant; Rx: seizures

N

Nabumetone (RELAFEN): NSAID analgesic; Rx: arthritis
Nadolol (CORGARD): beta blocker; Rx: HTN, angina
Nafcillin: penicillin antibiotic; Rx: bacterial infection
Naftifine (NAFTIN): topical antifungal agent
NAFTIN (naftifine): topical antifungal agent
Nalbuphine (NUBAIN): opioid agonist-antagonist analgesic; Rx: pain relief, pruritis
Naltrexone (REVIA): narcotic antagonist; Rx: narcotic or alcohol addiction
NAMENDA (memantine): NMDA antagonist; Rx: Alzheimer's disease
Naphazoline OPTH (NAPHCON): vasoconstrictor; Rx: relief of eye redness, irritation
NAPHCON OPTH (naphazoline): vasoconstrictor; Rx: relief of eye redness, irritation
NAPROSYN (naproxen): NSAID analgesic; Rx: arthritis, pain, inflammation, headache
NARDIL (phenelzine): MAO inhibitor; Rx: depression, bulimia
NASACORT AQ (triamcinolone): nasal corticosteroid; Rx: allergic rhinitis
NASALCROM (cromolyn): nasal anti-inflammatory agent; rhinitis
NASAREL (flunisolide): nasal corticosteroid; Rx: allergic rhinitis
NASONEX (mometasone): nasal corticosteroid; Rx: allergic rhinitis
NATRECOR (nesiritide): b-type natriuretic peptide vasodilator; Rx: CHF
NAVANE (thiothixene): antipsychotic; Rx: schizophrenia
NECON (ethinyl estradiol and norethindrone): contraceptive; Rx: prevent pregnancy, acne, menopause
Nefazodone (SERZONE): antidepressant; Rx: depression
Nelfinavir (VIRACEPT): protease inhibitor antiretroviral; Rx: HIV
NEMBUTAL (pentobarbital): barbiturate; Rx: insomnia, sleep induction, status epilepticus
Neomycin: aminoglycoside antibiotic; Rx: preoperative bowel preparation, encephalopathy
NEOPROFEN (ibuprofen lysine): Rx: closure patent ductus arteriosus in premature infants

NEORAL (cyclosporine): immunosuppressant, Rx: organ transplant

NEOSPORIN (neomycin/polymyxin/bacitracin): topical antibiotic compound, Rx: topical infections

NEPHROCAPS (vitamins): vitamin supplement, Rx: uremia, renal failure

NEULASTA (pegfilgrastim): colony stimulating factor, Rx: myelosuppressive chemotherapy

NEURONTIN (gabapentin): anticonvulsant, Rx: seizures, postherpetic neuralgia

NEUPOGEN (filgrastim): white blood cell stimulator, Rx: chemotherapy, bone marrow transplant

Nevirapine (VIRAMUNE): antiretroviral, Rx: HIV

NEXIUM (esomeprazole): protein pump inhibitor, Rx: esophagitis, GERD, ulcers

Niacin (vitamin B-3): nicotinic acid, Rx: hypercholesterolemia, hypertriglyceridemia

NIACOR (niacin): vitamin B-3, Rx: hypercholesterolemia, hypertriglyceridemia

NIASPAN (niacin slow release): vitamin B-3, Rx: hypercholesterolemia, hypertriglyceridemia

Nicardipine (CARDENE): calcium channel blocker, Rx: angina, HTN

NICODERM (transdermal nicotine): Rx: smoking cessation

NICOMIDE-T (niacinamide): vitamin, water soluable, Rx: pellagra, acne

NICORETTE (nicotine): smoking cessation aid, Rx: relief of nicotine withdrawal

Nicotinic Acid (niacin): vitamin B-3, Rx: hypercholesterolemia, hypertriglyceridemia

NICOTROL Inhaler (nicotine): Rx: smoking cessation

NICOTROL NS (nicotine): Rx: smoking cessation

Nifedipine (PROCARDIA, ADALAT): calcium channel blocker, Rx: angina, HTN

NIFEREX, NIFEREX-150 (iron): mineral, Rx: anemia

NILANDRON (nilutamide): antiandrogen, Rx: prostate cancer

Nimodipine (NIMOTOP): calcium channel blocker, Rx: improves neurological deficits after subarachnoid hemorrhage

NIMOTOP (nimodipine): calcium channel blocker, Rx: improves neurological deficits after subarachnoid hemorrhage

Nisoldipine (SULAR): calcium channel blocker, Rx: HTN

NITRO-DUR (nitroglycerin): transdermal nitrate, Rx: angina

Nitrofurantoin (macrandatin): antibacterial agent, Rx: UTI

Nitroglycerin (NITROSTAT): vasodilator, Rx: angina
NITROLINGUAL SPRAY (nitroglycerin): nitrate, Rx: angina
NITROMIST (nitroglycerin): vasodilator lingual spray, Rx: angina
NITROSTAT (nitroglycerin): vasodilator, Rx: angina
NIX (permethrin): parasiticide, Rx: head lice
Nizatidine (AXID): histamine-2 antagonist, Rx: ulcers, GERD
NIZORAL (ketoconazole): antifungal agent, Rx: fungal infections
NORCO (hydrocodone/APAP): narcotic analgesic compound, Rx: moderate to severe pain
NORDETTE (ethinyl estradiol and levonorgestrel): contraceptive, Rx: prevent pregnancy
NORFLEX (orphenadrine): skeletal muscle relaxant
Norfloxacin (NOROXIN): fluoroquinolone antibiotic, Rx: bacterial infections
NORGESIC (orphenadrine): skeletal muscle relaxant
NORINYL (ethinyl estradiol and norethindrone): contraceptive, Rx: prevent pregnancy, acne, menopause
NOROXIN (norfloxacin): fluoroquinolone antibiotic, Rx: bacterial infections
NORPACE, NORPACE CR (disopyramide): antiarrhythmic, Rx: ventricular dysrhythmias
NORPRAMIN (desipramine): a tricyclic antidepressant, Rx: depression
NOR-QD (norethindrone): contraceptive, Rx: amenorrhea, endometriosis, prevent pregnancy
NORTREL (ethinyl estradiol and norethindrone): contraceptive, Rx: prevent pregnancy, acne, menopause
Nortriptyline (PAMELOR): a tricyclic antidepressant
NORVASC (amlodipine): calcium blocker, Rx: HTN, angina
NORVIR (ritonavir): protease inhibitor antiretroviral, Rx: HIV
NOVANTRONE (mitoxantrone): antineoplastic, Rx: prostate cancer, leukemia, multiple sclerosis
NOVOLIN R (regular insulin): hypoglycemic, Rx: diabetes
NOVOLOG (insulin aspart): hypoglycemic, Rx: diabetes
NOVOLOG MIX 70/30 (insulin mixture): hypoglycemic, Rx: diabetes
NUBAIN (nalbuphine): opioid agonist-antagonist analgesic, Rx: pain relief, pruritis
NUVIGIL (armodafinil): CNS stimulant, Rx: narcolepsy, shift-work sleep disorder
Nystatin (MYCOSTATIN): antifungal, Rx: candidiasis
NYSTOP (nystatin): antifungal, Rx: candidiasis

O

Octreotide (SANDOSTATIN): antidiarrheal, growth inhibitor, Rx: acromegaly, diarrhea associated with carcinoid and intestinal tumors

OCUFLOX OPTH (ofloxacin): fluoroquinolone antibiotic, Rx: conjunctivitis, corneal ulcers

Ofloxacin (FLOXIN): fluoroquinolone antibiotic, Rx: bacterial infections

Olanzapine (ZYPREXA): antipsychotic, Rx: schizophrenia, bipolar disorder

Olopatadine (PATANOL): antihistamine, Rx: allergic conjunctivitis

Olsalazine (DIPENTUM): salicylate, Rx: ulcerative colitis

Omeprazole (PRILOSEC): suppresses gastric acid secretion, Rx: ulcers, esophagitis, GERD

OMNARIS (ciclesonide): intranasal steroid, Rx: allergic rhinitis

OMNICEF (cefdinir): cephalosporin antibiotic, Rx: bacterial infections

OMNIHIST LA (chlorpheniramine/phenylephrine/methscopalamine): antihistamine/decongestant, Rx: rhinitis, colds

Ondansetron (ZOFRAN): antinauseant, Rx: nausea and vomiting secondary to chemotherapy, radiation, and surgery

OPANA (oxymorphone): opioid analgesic, Rx: moderate to severe pain

Opium Tincture (morphine): opioid analgesic, Rx: diarrhea

OPTIVAR OPTH (azelastine): antihistamine, Rx: allergic conjunctivitis

ORAMORPH SR (morphine sulfate SR): opioid analgesic, Rx: moderate to severe pain

ORENCIA (abatacept): immunomodulator, Rx: rheumatoid arthritis

ORINASE (tolbutamide): oral hypoglycemic, Rx: diabetes (type 2)

Orphenadrine (NORFLEX): skeletal muscle relaxant

ORTHO EVRA (ethinyl estradiol and norelgestromin): contraceptive, Rx: prevent pregnancy

ORTHO TRI-CYCLEN (ethinyl estradiol and norgestimate): contraceptive, Rx: prevent pregnancy, acne

ORTHO-CEPT (ethinyl estradiol and desogestrel): contraceptive, Rx: prevent pregnancy

ORTHO-CYCLEN (ethinyl estradiol and norgestimate): contraceptive, Rx: prevent pregnancy, acne

ORTHO-EST (piperazine estrone sulfate): estrogen derivative, Rx: menopause, osteoporosis

158

ORTHO-NOVUM (ethinyl estradiol and norethindrone): contraceptive, Rx: prevent pregnancy, acne, menopause

OS-CAL (calcium, vitamin D): calcium salt, electrolyte supplement, Rx: antacid, dietary supplement

OVCON (ethinyl estradiol and norethindrone): contraceptive, Rx: prevent pregnancy, acne, menopause

OVIDE (malathon): antiparasitic/scabicidal agent, Rx: head lice and their ova

Oxacillin: penicillin class antibiotic, Rx: bacterial infections

Oxandrolone (OXANDRIN): anabolic steroid, Rx: osteoporosis, promotes weight gain

Oxaprozin (DAYPRO): NSAID analgesic, Rx: arthritis

Oxazepam (SERAX): benzodiazepine hypnotic, Rx: anxiety, alcohol withdrawal

Oxcarbazepine (TRILEPTAL): anticonvulsant, Rx: partial seizures

Oxiconazole (OXISTAT): topical antifungal, Rx: fungal infections

OXISTAT (oxiconazole): topical antifungal, Rx: fungal infections

OXSORALEN (methoxypsoralen): psoralen topical, Rx: repigmenting agent

Oxybutynin (DITROPAN): anticholinergic, antispasmodic, Rx: overactive bladder

Oxycodone (ROXICODNE, OXYCONTIN): opioid analgesic, Rx: moderate to severe pain

Oxycodone/ASA (PERCODAN): opioid analgesic/aspirin, Rx: moderate to severe pain

Oxycodone w/APAP (ENDOCET, PERCOCET, TYLOX): opioid analgesic/APAP, Rx: moderate to severe pain

OXYCONTIN (oxycodone SR): opioid analgesic, Rx: moderate to severe pain

OXYFAST (oxycodone): opioid analgesic, Rx: moderate to severe pain

Oxymetazoline (AFRIN): nasal decongestant, Rx: sinusitis, cold

Oxymetholone (ANADROL-50): anabolic steroid/androgen, Rx: anemia

Oxytocin (PITOCIN): stimulates uterine contractions, Rx: induction of labor

OXYTROL (oxybutynin): transdermal anticholinergic, antispasmodic, Rx: overactive bladder

PACERONE (amiodarone): antiarrhythmic, Rx: dysrhythmias

Paclitaxel (TAXOL): antineoplastic, Rx: ovarian cancer, breast cancer, Kaposi's sarcoma

Palivizumab (SYNAGIS): antiviral antibody, Rx: respiratory syncytial virus prevention

PAMELOR (nortriptyline): tricyclic antidepressant, Rx: depression

PANCREASE, PANCREASE MT (pancrelipase): pancreatic enzymes replacement, Rx: chronic pancreatitis, cystic fibrosis

Pancrelipase (CREON 5, PANCREASE): pancreatic enzymes replacement, Rx: chronic pancreatitis, cystic fibrosis

PANGESTYME (pancrelipase): pancreatic enzymes replacement, Rx: chronic pancreatitis, cystic fibrosis

Pantoprazole (PROTONIX): suppresses gastic acid, Rx: ulcers, GERD

PARAPLATIN (carboplatin): antineoplastic, Rx: ovarian cancer

PARCOPA (carbidopa/levodopa): dopamine precursors, Rx: Parkinson's disease

PAREGORIC (morphine): opioid analgesic, Rx: diarrhea

Paricalcitol (ZEMPLAR): vitamin D, Rx: hyperparathyroidism in chronic kidney disease

PARNATE (tranylcypromine): MAO inhibitor, Rx: depression

Paroxetine (PAXIL): SSRI antidepressant, Rx: depression, OCD, anxiety, PTSD

PASER (aminosalicylic acid): antibacterial, Rx: tuberculosis

PATANASE (olopatadine): nasal antihistamine, Rx: allergic rhinitis

PATANOL OPTH (olopatadine): antihistamine, Rx: allergic conjunctivitis

PAXIL (paroxetine): SSRI antidepressant, Rx: depression, OCD, anxiety, PTSD

PEDIAFLOR (fluoride): mineral, Rx: osteoporosis, dental caries

PEDIAPRED (prednisolone): glucocorticoid, Rx: allergies, arthritis, multiple sclerosis

PEDI-DRI (nystatin): topical antifungal antibiotic, Rx: fungal infection

PEGANONE (ethotoin): anticonvulsant, Rx: seizures

PEGASYS (peginterferon alfa-2a): interferon, Rx: chronic hepatitis B and C

PEGINTRON (interferon alfa-2b): antiviral, Rx: chronic hepatitis C

Pemirolast OPTH (ALAMAST). anti-inflammatory, Rx: allergic conjunctivitis

Pemoline (CYLERT): stimulant, Rx: ADHD

Penbutolol (LEVATOL): beta blocker, Rx: HTN

Penciclovir (DENAVIR): topical antiviral, Rx: herpes, cold sores

Penicillamine (CUPRIMINE, DEPEN): chelator, antirheumatic, Rx: heavy metal poisoning, Wilson's disease, arthritis, cystinuria

Penicillin (VEETIDS): penicillin antibiotic, Rx: bacterial infection

Pentamidine (PENTAM 300): antiprotozoal, Rx: P. carinii pneumonia

PENTASA (mesalamine): anti-inflammatory, Rx: ulcerative colitis

Pentazocine (TALWIN): opioid agonist-antagonist analgesic, Rx: moderate to severe pain

Pentazocine/Naloxone (TALWIN NX): opioid analgesic compound, Rx: pain

Pentazocine/APAP (TALACEN): opioid analgesic/APAP compound

Pentobarbital (NEMBUTAL): barbiturate hypnotic, Rx: insomnia, status epilepticus

Pentostatin (NIPENT): antineoplastic, Rx: hairy cell leukemia

Pentoxifylline (TRENTAL): reduces blood viscosity, Rx: intermittent claudication

PEPCID, PEPCID AC (famotidine): histamine-2 blocker, reduces gastric acid, Rx: ulcers, GERD

PERCOCET (oxycodone/APAP): opioid analgesic, Rx: moderate to severe pain

PERCODAN (oxycodone/aspirin): opioid analgesic, Rx: moderate to severe pain

PERFOROMIST (formoterol): beta$_2$ adenergic agonist, long acting, Rx: asthma, COPD

PERIACTIN (cyproheptadine): antihistamine, Rx: allergies

PERI-COLACE (docusate/senna): stool softener/laxative, Rx: constipation

Perindopril (ACEON): ACE inhibitor, Rx: HTN, CAD

Permethrin (ELIMITE, ACTICIN, NIX): parasiticide, Rx: head lice, scabies

Perphenazine (TRILAFON): anitpsychotic, Rx: schizophrenia, hiccoughs

PERSANTINE (dipyridamole): platelet inhibitor, Rx: blood clots after heart valve replacement

Phenazopyridine (PYRIDIUM): urinary tract analgesic, Rx: relief of pain on urination

Phenelzine (NARDIL): MAO inhibitor, Rx: depression

PHENERGAN (promethazine): sedative/antiemetic, Rx: rhinitis, urticaria, nausea and vomiting

Phenobarbital: barbiturate sedative, Rx: sedative, anticonvulsant

Phentermine (ADIPEX-P): amphetamine, Rx: obesity

Phenyl Salicylate/methenamine (PROSED/DS, UROGESIC BLUE): analgesic, Rx: urinary tract discomfort, cystitis, urethritis

Phenylephrine (NEO-SYNEPHRINE, SUDAFED PE): decongestant, Rx: colds, allergies

Phenytoin (DILANTIN): anticonvulsant, Rx: epilepsy

PHISOHEX (hexachlorophene): bacteriostatic skin cleanser

PhosLo (calcium): antidote, calcium salt, phosphate binder, Rx: hyperphosphatemia

PHRENILIN, PHRENILIN FORTE (butalbital/acetaminophen): barbiturate sedative, analgesic, Rx: tension headache

Phytonadione (AQUAMEPHYTON): vitamin K1, Rx: coagulation disorders

Pilocarpine (SALAGEN): cholinergic, Rx: dry mouth, Sjogren's syndrome

Pilocarpine OPTH (ISOPTO CARPINE, PILOCAR): cholinergic miotic, Rx: glaucoma

PIMA (potassium iodide): expectorant, Rx: asthma, bronchitis

Pindolol (VISKEN): beta blocker, Rx: HTN

Pioglitazone (ACTOS): oral hypoglycemic, Rx: diabetes (type 2)

Piperacillin (PIPRACIL): penicillin antibiotic, Rx: bacterial infections

Pirbuterol (MAXAIR): beta bronchodilator, Rx: asthma, COPD

Piroxicam (FELDENE): NSAID analgesic, Rx: arthritis

PLAQUENIL (hydroxychloroquine): antimalarial agent, Rx: malaria, rheumatoid arthritis, lupus

PLAVIX (clopidogrel): platelet inhibitor, Rx: MI, stroke, atherosclerosis

PLETAL (cilostazol): platelet inhibitor, Rx: intermittent claudication

PNEUMOTUSSIN (guaifenesin/hydrocodone): expectorant/opioid antitussive, Rx: cough

PODOCON-25 (podophyllin): cytotoxic, Rx: genital warts

Podofilox (CONDYLOX): destroys warts, Rx: anogenital warts

Podophyllin (PODOCON-25): cytotoxic agent, Rx: genital warts

Polyethylene glycol (MIRALAX): osmotic laxative, Rx: constipation

Polymyxin B (Poly-Rx) polymixin B sulfate, antibiotic, Rx: acute infections

POLYTRIM OPTH (trimethoprim/polymyxin): antibiotic compound, Rx: eye infections

PONSTEL (mefenamic acid): NSAID analgesic, Rx: mild to moderate pain

Posaconazole (NOXAFIL): antifungal, Rx: fungal infections

Potassium citrate (UROCIT-K): urinary alkalinizer, Rx: kidney stones

Potassium iodide (PIMA): expectorant, Rx: asthma, bronchitis

Pramipexole (MIRAPEX): dopamine agonist, Rx: Parkinson's disease, restless leg syndrome

PRAMOSONE (hydrocortisone/pramoxine): topical corticosteroid/anesthetic compound, Rx: dermatoses

Pramoxine (PRAX, SARNA): topical anesthetic, Rx: relief of itching, pain

PRANDIMET (repaglinide/metformin): oral hypoglycemics, Rx: diabetes (type 2)

PRANDIN (repaglinide): oral hypoglycemia, Rx: diabetes (type 2)

PRAVACHOL (pravastatin): statin, Rx: hypercholesterolemia, CAD

Pravastatin (PRAVACHOL): statin, Rx: hypercholesterolemia, CAD

PRAX (pramoxine): topical anesthetic, Rx: relief of itching, pain

Prazosin (MINIPRESS): alpha-1 blocker, vasodilator, Rx: HTN

PRECOSE (acarbose): delays carbohydrate digestion, Rx: diabetes mellitus (type 2)

Prednisolone (ORAPRED, PRELONE): glucocorticoid, Rx: adrenal insufficiency, allergies, RA, lupus, COPD

Prednisone (DELTASONE): glucocorticoid, Rx: adrenal insufficiency, allergies, RA, lupus, COPD

PRELONE (prednisolone): glucocorticoid, Rx: adrenal insufficiency, allergies, RA, lupus, COPD

PREMARIN (conjugated estrogens): hormones, Rx: menopause

PREMPRO (estrogens/progesterone): hormones, Rx: menopause

PREVACID (lansoprazole): gastric acid pump inhibitor, Rx: ulcers, esophagitis, GERD

PREVPAC (lansoprazole/amoxicillin/clarithromycin): H. Pylori treatment, Rx: duodenal ulcers

PRIFTIN (rifapentine): antibiotic, Rx: tuberculosis

PRILOSEC (omeprazole): gastric acid pump inhibitor, Rx: ulcers, esophagitis, GERD

Primaquine: antimalarial agent, Rx: malaria

PRIMATENE MIST (epinephrine): alpha/beta agonist, Rx: bronchospasms, asthma

PRIMAXIN (imipenem/cilastatin): carbapenem antibiotic, Rx: bacterial infections

Primidone (MYSOLINE): anticonvulsant, Rx: seizures

PRINIVIL (lisinopril): ACE inhibitor, Rx: HTN, CHF

PRINZIDE (lisinopril/HCTZ): ACE inhibitor/diuretic, Rx: HTN

PRISTIQ (desvenlafaxine): antidepressant, Rx: depression

PROAMATINE (midodrine): vasopressor, Rx: orthostatic hypotension

PRO-BANTHINE (propantheline): anticholinergic, inhibits gastric acid secretion, Rx: peptic ulcers

Probenecid: increases uric acid secretion, Rx: gout

Procainamide (PROCANBID): antiarrhythmic, Rx: dysrhythmias

PROCANBID (procainamide): antiarrhythmic, Rx: dysrhythmias

Procarbazine (MATULANE): antineoplastic, Rx: Hodgkin's disease

PROCARDIA, PROCARDIA XL (nifedipine): calcium channel blocker, Rx: angina, HTN

Prochlorperazine (COMPAZINE): phenothiazine antiemetic, Rx: nausea and vomiting, anxiety

PROCRIT (epoetin alfa): stimulates red blood cell production, Rx: anemia, in renal failure, HIV, and chemotherapy

PROCTOCORT (hydrocortisone): rectal corticosteroid, Rx: ulcerative colitis

PROCTOCREAM-HC (hydrocortisone/pramoxine): topical corticosteroid/anesthetic compound, Rx: dermatoses

PROCTOFOAM-HC (hydrocortisone): steroid anti-inflammatory, Rx: inflammation, itching

Progesterone (PROMETRIUM): progestin, Rx: endometrial hyperplasia, secondary amenorrhea

PROGRAF (tacrolimus): immunosuppressant, Rx: transplant

PROLASTIN (alpha-1 proteinase inhibitor): Rx: alpha-1 antitrypsin deficiency, emphysema

Promethazine (PHENERGAN): phenothiazine, Rx: rhinitis, allergic conjunctivitis, sedation, nausea and vomiting

PROMETRIUM (progesterone): progestin, Rx: endometrial hyperplasia, secondary amenorrhea

Propafenone (RYTHMOL): beta blocker, antiarrhythmic, Rx: PSVT, paroxysmal atrial fibrillation

Propantheline: anticholinergic, inhibits gastric acid secretion, Rx: peptic ulcers

Proparacaine OPTH (ALCAINE): anesthetic, Rx: corneal anesthesia

PROPECIA (finasteride): 5-alpha-reductase inhibitor, Rx: hair loss, men only

Propoxyphene (DARVON): opioid analgesic, Rx: mild to moderate pain

Propoxyphene/APAP (DARVON): opioid analgesic, Rx: mild to moderate pain

Propranolol (INDERAL): beta blocker, Rx: HTN, prophylaxis of: angina, cardiac dysrhythmias, AMI, migraine headache

Propylthiouracil: antithyroid, Rx: hyperthyroidism

PROSCAR (finasteride): antiandrogen, Rx: benign prostatic hypertrophy

PROSED/DS (methenamine/phenyl salicylate/methylene blue/benzoic acid/hyoscyamine): bactericidal, analgesic, antiseptic, Rx: urinary tract infections

PROSOM (estazolam): benzodiazepine hypnotic, Rx: insomnia

PROTONIX (pantoprazole): proton pump inhibitor, Rx: ulcers, GERD

PROTOPAM (pralidoxime): anticholinergic, Rx: organophosphate poisoning

PROVENTIL, PROVENTIL HFA (albuterol): beta$_2$ agonist bronchodilator, Rx: COPD, asthma

PROVERA (medroxyprogesterone): hormone, Rx: amenorrhea, irregular vaginal bleeding

PROVIGIL (modafinil): stimulant, Rx: narcolepsy, daytime sleepiness

PROZAC (fluoxetine): a heterocyclic antidepressant

Pseudoephedrine (SUDAFED): decongestant, Rx: colds, allergies

PSORCON E (diflorasone): topical corticosteroid, Rx: dermatoses

Psyllium (KONSYL, METAMUCIL): fiber laxative, Rx: constipation

PULMICORT (budesonide): inhaled corticosteroid, Rx: asthma

PULMOZYME (dornase alfa): lytic enzyme, dissolves lung secretions, Rx: cystic fibrosis

PURINETHOL (mercaptopurine): antineplastic, Rx: leukemia

Pyrazinamide: antibacterial, Rx: tuberculosis

PYRIDIUM (phenazopyridine): urinary tract analgesic, Rx: relief of pain on urination

Pyridostigmine (MESTINON): anticholinesterase, Rx: myasthenia gravis

Pyridoxine (vitamin B6): vitamin

Pyrimethamine (DARAPRIM): antiparasitic, Rx: toxoplasmosis, malaria

Q

QUALAQUIN (quinine): antimalarial, Rx: malaria
QUESTRAN (cholestyramine): bile acid sequestrant,
Rx: antihyperlipidemic
Quetiapine (SEROQUEL): antipsychotic, Rx: schizophrenia,
bipolar disorder
Quinapril (ACCUPRIL): ACE inhibitor, Rx: HTN, CHF
Quinapril/HCTZ (QUINARETIC, ACCURETIC): ACE inhibitor/
diuretic, Rx: HTN
QUINARETIC (quinapril/HCTZ): ACE inhibitor/diuretic, Rx: HTN
Quinidine: antiarrhythmic, Rx: atrial fibrillation/flutter, malaria
Quinine: antimalarial, Rx: malaria
Quinupristin/Dalfopristin (SYNERCID): streptogramin antibiotic,
Rx: bacterial infections
QUIXIN OPTH (levofloxacin): fluoroquinolone, Rx: conjunctivitis
QVAR (beclomethasone): inhaled corticosteroid, Rx: asthma

R

Raloxifene (EVISTA): estrogen modulator, Rx: osteoporosis,
breast cancer prevention
Ramipril (ALTACE): ACE inhibitor, Rx: HTN, CHF post MI
RANEXA (ranolazine): anti-ischemic, Rx: chronic angina
Ranitidine (ZANTAC): histamine-2 blocker, Rx: ulcers, GERD,
esophagitis
RAPAFLO (silodosin): alpha receptor agonist, Rx: benign prostatic
hyperplasia
RAPAMUNE (sirolimus): immunosuppressive, Rx: renal transplant
RAPTIVA (efalizumab): immunosuppressant, Rx: psoriasis
RAZADYNE (galantamine): acetylcholinesterase inhibitor,
Rx: Alzheimer's disease
REBETOL (ribavirin): antiviral, Rx: hepatitis C
REBETRON (interferon alfa/ribavirin): antivirals, Rx: hepatitis C
Rebif (interferon-beta-1a): immunomodulator, Rx: multiple sclerosis
RECOMBINATE (Factor VIII): antihemophilic factor, Rx: hemophilia
REFLUDAN (lepirudin): anticoagulant, Rx: heparin induced
thrombocytopenia
REGLAN (metoclopramide): improves gastric emptying,
Rx: heartburn, diabetic gastroparesis

RELAFEN (nabumetone): NSAID analgesic, Rx: arthritis
RELENZA (zanamivir): antiviral, Rx: influenza
RELISTOR (methylnaltrexone): GI tract opioid antagonist, Rx: opioid induced constipation
RELPAX (eletriptan): serotonin receptor agonist, Rx: migraine headaches
REMERON (mirtazapine): antidepressant, Rx: depression
REMICADE (infliximab): neutralizes tumor necrosis factor, Rx: Crohn's disease, arthritis, ulcerative colitis, psoriasis
RENAGEL (sevelamer): phosphate binder, Rx: hyperphosphatemia in renal disease
REQUIP (ropinirole): dopaminergic, Rx: Parkinson's disease, restless legs syndrome
RESCRIPTOR (delavirdine): antiretroviral, Rx: HIV
RESTASIS OPTH (cyclosporine): immunomodulator, Rx: increases tear production
RESTORIL (temazepam): benzodiazepine hypnotic, Rx: insomnia
RETEVASE (reteplase): thrombolytic, Rx: AMI
RETIN A (tretinoin): retinoid, Rx: acne
RETROVIR (zidovudine): antiretroviral agent, Rx: HIV
REVATIO (sildenafil): vasodilator, Rx: pulmonary artery hypertension
REYATAZ (atazanavir): antiretroviral, Rx: HIV
RHINOCORT (budesonide): nasal corticosteroid, Rx: allergic rhinitis
Ribavirin (REBETOL): antiviral, Rx: hepatitis C
RIFADIN (rifampin): antibiotic, Rx: tuberculosis, prophylaxis for N. meningitidis
RIFAMATE (rifampin/isoniazid): antibiotics, Rx: tuberculosis
Rifampin (RIFADIN): antibiotic, Rx: tuberculosis, prophylaxis for N. meningitidis
Rifapentine (PRIFTIN): antibiotic, Rx: tuberculosis
RIFATER (isoniazid/rifampin/pyrazinamide): antibiotic, Rx: tuberculosis
Rifaximin (XIFAXAN): antibiotic, Rx: traveler's diarrhea, hepatic encephalopathy
Rimantadine (FLUMADINE): antiviral, Rx: influenza A virus
RIOMET (metformin): oral hypoglycemic, Rx: diabetes (type 2)
Risedronate (ACTONEL): bone stabilizer, Rx: Paget's disease, osteoporosis
RISPERDAL (risperidone): antipsychotic, Rx: schizophrenia, autism, bipolar disorder

Risperidone (RISPERDAL): antipsychotic, Rx: schizophrenia, autism, bipolar disorder

RITALIN (methylphenidate): stimulant, Rx: attention deficit hyperactivity disorder in children, narcolepsy

Ritonavir (NORVIR): antiretroviral, Rx: HIV

RITUXAN (rituximab): antineoplastic, Rx: non-Hodgkin lymphoma, RA

Rivastigmine (EXELON): cholinesterase inhibitor, Rx: dementia in Alzheimer's disease and Parkinson's disease

ROBAXIN (methocarbamol): skeletal muscle relaxant

ROBINUL, **ROBINUL FORTE** (glycopyrrolate): anticholinergic, Rx: peptic ulcers

ROBITUSSIN (guaifenesin): expectorant

ROCALTROL (calcitrol): vitamin D analog, Rx: hypocalcemia in renal disease, hypoparathyroidism, bone disease

ROCEPHIN (ceftriaxone): cephalosporin antibiotic, Rx: bacterial infections

Ropinirole (REQUIP): dopaminergic, Rx: Parkinson's disease, restless leg syndrome

Rosiglitazone (AVANDIA): oral hypoglycemic, Rx: diabetes (type 2)

ROWASA (mesalamine): anti-inflammatory, Rx: colitis, proctitis

ROXANOL (morphine): opioid analgesic, Rx: moderate to severe pain

ROXICET (oxycodone/APAP): opioid analgesic, Rx: moderate to severe pain

ROXICODONE (oxycodone): opioid analgesic, Rx: moderate to severe pain

ROZEREM (ramelteon): melatonin agonist, Rx: insomnia

RYNATAN (phenylephrine/chlorpheniramine/pyrilamine): antihistamine/decongestant compound, Rx: common cold

RYNATUSS: antitussive/decongestant/antihistamine, Rx: common cold

RYTHMOL, **RYTHMOL SR** (propafenone): antiarrhythmic, Rx: PSVT, paroxysmal atrial fibrillation

S

SALAGEN (pilocarpine): cholinergic, Rx: dry mouth

SALIVART: saliva substitute, Rx: dry mouth

Salmeterol (SEREVENT): inhaled beta$_2$ bronchodilator, Rx: asthma, COPD

SAL-PLANT Gel (salicylic acid): for removal of common warts

Salsalate: NSAID analgesic, Rx: arthritis

SANDIMMUNE (cyclosporine): immunosuppressant agent, Rx: organ transplants

SANDOSTATIN (octreotide): antidiarrheal, growth inhibitor, Rx: acromegaly, diarrhea associated with carcinoid and intestinal tumors

Saquinavir (INVIRASE): antiretroviral, Rx: HIV

SARAFEM (fluoxetine): antidepressant, Rx: premenstrual dysphoric disorder

SAVELLA (milnacipran): selective serotonin/norepinephrine inhibitor, Rx: fibromyalgia

Scopolamine: anticholinergic, Rx: motion sickness, IBS, diverticulitis

SECONAL (secobarbital): barbiturate hypnotic, Rx: insomnia

SECTRAL (acebutolol): beta blocker, Rx: HTN, angina, dysrhythmias

Selegiline (ELDEPRYL): MAO inhibitor, Rx: Parkinson's disease

SEMPREX-D (acrivastine/pseudoephedrine): antihistamine/decongestant, Rx: allergic rhinitis

Senna Extract (SENOKOT): laxative, Rx: constipation

SENNA-S, SENOKOT-S (senna/docusate): laxative/stool softener, Rx: constipation

SENOKOT, SENOKOT XTRA (senna): laxative, Rx: constipation

SENSIPAR (cinacalcet): reduces PTH levels, Rx: 2nd hyperparathyroidism in dialysis patients

SEPTRA, SEPTRA DS (trimethoprim/sulfamethoxazole): sulfa antibacterial compound, Rx: bacterial infections

SEREVENT (salmeterol): inhaled beta$_2$ bronchodilator, Rx: asthma, COPD

SEROQUEL (quetiapine): antipsychotic, Rx: schizophrenia, bipolar disorder

SEROSTIM (somatropin): hormone, Rx: AIDS wasting

Sertraline (ZOLOFT): antidepressant, Rx: depression, panic disorder, obsessive-compulsive disorder, premenstrual dysphoric disorder

SERZONE (nefazodone): antidepressant, Rx: depression

SILVADENE (silver sulfadiazine): topical antimicrobial agent, Rx: burn wounds

SIMCOR (niacin/simvastatin): cholesterol reducers, Rx: hypercholesterolemia, hypertriglyceridemia

Simethicone (MYLICON): Rx: relief of excess gas in GI tract

SIMPLY COUGH LIQUID (dextromethorphan): antitussive, Rx: cough

Simvastatin (Zocor): statin, Rx: hypercholesterolemia, CAD

SINEMET CR (carbidopa/levodopa): dopamine precursors, Rx: Parkinson's disease

SINEQUAN (doxepin): tricyclic antidepressant, Rx: depression, anxiety

SINGULAIR (montelukast): leukotriene receptor antagonist, Rx: asthma, allergic rhinitis

SINUVENT (phenylephrine/guaifenesin): decongestant/expectorant, Rx: sinusitis, rhinitis

Sirolimus (RAPAMUNE): immunosuppressive, Rx: renal transplant

SKELAXIN (metaxalone): skeletal muscle relaxant

SLO-NIACIN (niacin CR): Rx: hypercholesterolemia, hypertriglyceridemia

Sodium polysterene sulfonate (KAYEXALATE): Na/K exchange resin, Rx: hyperkalemia

SOMA (carisoprodol): muscle relaxant, Rx: muscle spasm

SONATA (zaleplon): hypnotic, Rx: insomnia

SORIATANE (acitretin): retinoid, Rx: psoriasis

Sotalol (BETAPACE): antiarrhythmic, Rx: dysrhythmias

SPECTAZOLE (econazole): topical antifungal agent

SPECTRACEF (cefditoren): cephalosporin antibiotic, Rx: bacterial infections

SPIRIVA (tiotropium): inhaled anticholinergic bronchodilator, Rx: COPD

Spironolactone (ALDACTONE): potassium-sparing diuretic, Rx: hyperaldosteronism, HTN, CHF

SPORANOX (itraconazole): antifungal, Rx: fungal infections

SSKI (potassium iodide): expectorant, Rx: asthma, bronchitis

STADOL NS (butorphanol): opioid agonist/antagonist analgesic, Rx: pain

STAGESIC (hydrocodone and acetaminophen): analgesic combination (opioid), Rx: pain

STALEVO (levodopa/carbidopa/entacapone): dopamine precursors, Rx: Parkinson's disease

STARLIX (nateglinide): oral hypoglycemic, Rx: diabetes (type 2)

STATUSS DM (dextromethorphan, phenylephrine, chlorpheniramine): non-narcotic antitussive, decongestant, antihistamine compound

Stavudine d4T (ZERIT): antiretroviral, Rx: HIV

STELAZINE (trifluoperazine): antipsychotic, Rx: schizophrenia

STRATTERA (atomoxetine): psychotherapeutic agent, Rx: ADHD
Streptomycin: aminoglycoside antibiotic, Rx: tuberculosis
STRIANT (testosterone): androgen, Rx: adult male hypogonadism
STROMECTOL (ivermectin): anti-parasite, Rx: intestinal nematodes
SUBOXONE (buprenorphine/naloxone): opioid analgesic/antagonist, Rx: opiate addiction
SUBUTEX (buprenorphine): narcotic analgesic, Rx: opiate addiction
Sucralfate (CARAFATE): anti-ulcer agent, Rx: duodenal ulcers
Sufentanil (SUFENTA): analgesic, opioid, general anesthetic, Rx: analgesic supplement
SULAR (nisoldipine): calcium channel blocker, Rx: HTN
Sulfacetamide OPTH (BLEPH-10): antibiotic, Rx: ocular infections
Sulfamethoxazole (SEPTRA): sulfa antibiotic, Rx: bacterial infections
Sulfamylon (MAFENIDE): topical antibiotic, Rx: burn wounds
Sulfasalazine (AZULFIDINE): anti-inflammatory, Rx: ulcerative colitis, rheumatoid arthritis
Sulfisoxazole (GANTRISIN): sulfonamide antibiotic, Rx: bacterial infections
Sulindac (CLINORIL): NSAID analgesic, Rx: arthritis
Sumatriptan (IMITREX): selective serotonin receptor agonist, Rx: migraine headache
SUPRAX (cefixime): cephalosporin antibiotic, Rx: bacterial infections
SURVANTA (beractant): lung surfactant in premature infants
SUSTIVA (efavirenz): antiretroviral, Rx: HIV
SYMBICORT (budesonide/formoterol): inhaled corticosteroid/beta$_2$ agonist, Rx: asthma, COPD
SYMBYAX (olanzapine/fluoxetine): antipsychotic/SSRI, Rx: bipolar disorder, resistant depression
SYMMETREL (amantadine): antiparkinson/antiviral, Rx: influenza A, Parkinson's disease
SYNAGIS (palivizumab): antiviral antibody, Rx: respiratory syncytial virus (prevention)
SYNAREL (naferelin): nasal gonadotropin-releasing hormone, Rx: endometriosis, precocious puberty
SYNERCID (quinupristin/dalfopristin): streptogramin antibiotic, Rx: bacterial infections
SYNTHROID (levothyroxine): thyroid hormone, Rx: hypothyroidism

T

TABLOID (thioguanine): antineoplastic, Rx: leukemia

TAGAMET (cimetidine): inhibits gastric acid secretion, Rx: ulcers

TALACEN (pentazocine/APAP): opioid agonist/antagonist analgesic/APAP, Rx: pain

TALWIN NX (pentazocine/naloxone): opioid agonist/antagonist analgesic, Rx: pain

TAMBOCOR (flecainide): antiarrhythmic, Rx: PSVT, paroxysmal atrial fibrillation

TAMIFLU (oseltamivir): antiviral, Rx: influenza

Tamoxifen: antiestrogen, Rx: breast cancer

TAPAZOLE (methimazole): antithyroid, Rx: hyperthyroidism

TARKA (trandolapril/verapamil): ACE inhibitor/calcium channel blocker, Rx: HTN

TASMAR (tolcapone): antiparkinson agent, COMT inhibitor, Rx: Parkinson's disease

TEGRETOL, TEGRETOL XR (carbamazepine): anticonvulsant, Rx: seizures, trigeminal neuralgia

TEKTURNA (Aliskeren): direct renin inhibitor, Rx: HTN

Telmisartan (MICARDIS): angiotensin II receptor agonist, Rx: HTN

Temazepam (RESTORIL): benzodiazepine hypnotic, Rx: insomnia

TEMOVATE (clobetasol): topical steroid anti-inflammatory, Rx: dermatoses

TENEX (guanfacine): centrally acting alpha agonist, Rx: HTN

TENORETIC (atenolol/Chlorthalidone): beta blocker/diuretic, Rx: HTN

TENORMIN (atenolol): beta blocker, Rx: hypertension, angina, MI

TENUATE (diethylpropion): stimulant, appetite suppressant, Rx: obesity

Terazosin (HYTRIN): alpha-1 blocker, Rx: HTN, benign prostatatic hyperplasia

Terbinafine (LAMISIL): antifungal, Rx: nail fungus, ringworm

Terbutaline (BRETHINE): beta$_2$ agonist bronchodilator, Rx: asthma, COPD

Terconazole (TERAZOL): antifungal, Rx: vaginal candidiasis

TESSALON (benzonatate): antitussive, Rx: cough

Testosterone (ANDRODERM, DEPO-TESTOSTERONE): androgen, Rx: hypogonadism

TESTRED (methyltestosterone): androgen, Rx: hypogonadism

Tetracycline (SUMYCIN): tetracycline antibiotic, Rx: bacterial infections

TEVETEN (eprosartan): angiotensin II receptor inhibitor, Rx: HTN

Thalidomide (THALOMID): immunosuppressant, Rx: HIV, leprosy

THALOMID (thalidomide): immunosuppressant, Rx: HIV, leprosy

THEO-24 (theophylline): bronchodilator, Rx: asthma, COPD
THEOCRON (theophylline): bronchodilator, Rx: asthma, COPD
Theophylline (THEO-24, UNIPHYL): bronchodilator, Rx: asthma, COPD
THERA-GESIC (salicylate): topical NSAID analgesic, Rx: arthritis
Thiamin: vitamin B1, Rx: thiamin deficiency
Thioridazine: antipsychotic, Rx: schizophrenia
Thiothixene (NAVANE): antipsychotic, Rx: schizophrenia
THORAZINE (chlorpromazine): antipsychotic, Rx: schizophrenia
Thyroid (ARMOUR THYROID): thyroid hormone, Rx: hypothyroidism
THYROLAR (liotrix): thyroid hormone, Rx: hypothyroidism
Tiagabine (GABITRIL): anticonvulsant, Rx: partial seizures
TIAZAC (diltiazem): calcium channel blocker, Rx: HTN, angina
Ticarcillin/clavulanate (TIMENTIN): penicillin antibiotic, Rx: bacterial infections
TICLID (ticlopidine): platelet inhibitor, Rx: stroke prophylaxis
Ticlodipine (TICLID): platelet inhibitor, Rx: stroke prophylaxis
TIGAN (trimethobenzamide): antiemetic, Rx: postoperative nausea and vomiting
TIKOSYN (dofetilide): antiarrhythmic, Rx: atrial fibrillation
TIMENTIN (ticarcillin/clavulanate): penicillin class antibiotic, Rx: bacterial infections
Timolol (BLOCADREN): beta blocker, Rx: HTN, MI, migraine
TIMOPTIC OPTH (timolol): beta blocker, Rx: glaucoma
TINACTIN (tolnaftate): topical antifungal, Rx: athlete's foot, jock itch
Tizanidine (ZANAFLEX): skeletal muscle relaxant
TOBI Solution Inhalation (tobramycin): aminoglycoside antibiotic, Rx: cystic fibrosis
TOBRADEX (tobramycin/dexamethasone): antibiotic/steroid, Rx: eye infection/inflammation
Tobramycin: aminoglycoside antibiotic, Rx: bacterial infections
TOBREX OPTH (tobramycin): aminoglycoside antibiotic, Rx: ocular infections
TOFRANIL, TOFRANIL PM (imipramine): tricyclic antidepressant, Rx: depression, anxiety
Tolazamide: oral hypoglycemic, Rx: diabetes (type 2)
Tolbutamide: oral hypoglycemic, Rx: diabetes (type 2)
Tolmetin: NSAID analgesic, Rx: arthritis
Tolnaftate (TINACTIN): topical antifungal, Rx: athlete's foot, jock itch

Tolterodine (DETROL): urinary bladder antispasmodic, Rx: overactive bladder

TOPAMAX (topiramate): anticonvulsant, Rx: seizures, migraine

TOPROL-XL (metoprolol): cardioselective beta blocker, Rx: HTN, angina, CHF

TORADOL (ketorolac): NSAID analgesic, Rx: acute pain

Torsemide (DEMADEX): loop diuretic, Rx: HTN, edema in CHF, kidney disease, liver disease

TOVIAZ (fesoterodine): anticholinergic, Rx: overactive bladder

TRACLEER (bosentan): endothelin receptor antagonist, Rx: pulmonary hypertension

Tramadol (ULTRAM): opioid analgesic, Rx: moderate to severe pain

TRANDATE (labetalol): beta blocker, Rx: hypertension

Trandolapril (MAVIK): ACE inhibitor, Rx: HTN, CHF post MI

TRANSDERM-SCOP (scopolamine): anticholinergic antiemetic, Rx: motion sickness prophylaxis

TRANXENE (clorazepate): benzodiazepine hypnotic, Rx: anxiety, seizures

TRAVATAN OPTH (travoprost): prostaglandin agonist, Rx: glaucoma

Trazodone: antidepressant, Rx: depression, insomnia

TRECATOR (ethionamide): antibiotic, Rx: tuberculosis

TRENTAL (pentoxifylline): reduces blood viscosity, Rx: intermittent claudication

Tretinoin (ATRALIN): retinoic acid derivative, topical, Rx: acne, skin care

Triamcinolone (KENALOG): topical corticosteroid, Rx: dermatoses

Triamcinolone (AZMACORT): inhaled corticosteroid, Rx: asthma

Triamterene/HCTZ (DYAZIDE, Maxzide): diuretics, Rx: HTN, water retention

Triazolam (HALCION): benzodiazepine hypnotic, Rx: insomnia

TRICOR (fenofibrate): lipid regulator, Rx: hyperlipidemia

Trifluoperazine (STELAZINE): antipsychotic, Rx: schizophrenia

TRIGLIDE (fenofibrate): lipid reducer, Rx: hyperlipidemia

Trihexyphenidyl (ARTANE): anticholinergic, Rx: Parkinson's disease

TRILEPTAL (oxcarbazepine): anticonvulsant, Rx: partial seizures

Trimethoprim: antibiotic, Rx: UTI

Trimethoprim/Sulfamethoxazole (BACTRIM, SEPTRA): sulfa antibiotic compound, Rx: bacterial infections

TRINESSA (ethinyl estradiol and norgestimate): contraceptive, Rx: prevent pregnancy, acne

TRI-NORINYL (ethinyl estradiol and norethindrone): contraceptive, Rx: prevent pregnancy, acne, menopause

TRIPHASIL (ethinyl estradiol and levonorgestrel): contraceptive, Rx: prevent pregnancy

TRIZIVIR (abacavir/lamivudine/zidovudine): antiretrovirals, Rx: HIV infection, hepatitis B

TRUSOPT OPTH (dorzolamide): decreases intraocular pressure Rx: glaucoma

TRUVADA (emtricitabine/tenofovir): antiretrovirals, Rx: HIV

TUSSAFED HC (hydrocodone/phenylephrine/guaifenesin): opioid antitussive/decongestant/expectorant

TUSSI-ORGANIDIN (guaifenesin/codeine): expectorant/opioid antitussive, Rx: cough

TUSSIONEX (hydrocodone/chlorpheniramine): opioid antitussive/ antihistamine, Rx: coughs, allergies, cold

TYGACIL (tigecycline): glycylcycline antibiotic, Rx: bacterial infections

TYKERB (lapatinib): antineoplastic agent, Rx: breast cancer

TYLENOL w/Codeine (APAP, codeine): opioid with APAP analgesic, Rx: mild to moderate pain

TYLENOL SINUS CONGESTION (phenylephrine/guaifenesin/APAP): decongestant/expectorant/analgesic, Rx: sinusitis, rhinitis, colds

TYZEKA (telbivudine): antiviral, Rx: hepatitis B

U

ULORIC (febuxostat): xanthine oxidase inhibitor, Rx: gout

ULTRACET (tramadol/APAP): opioid analgesic compound, Rx: acute pain

ULTRAM (tramadol): opioid analgesic, Rx: moderate to severe pain

ULTRASE, ULTRASE MT (pancrelipase): pancreatic enzymes replacement, Rx: chronic pancreatitis, cystic fibrosis

ULTRAVATE (halobetasol): topical corticosteroid, Rx: dermatoses

UNIPHYL (theophylline): bronchodilator, Rx: asthma, COPD

UNIRETIC (moexipril/HCTZ): ACE inhibitor/diuretic, Rx: HTN

UNISOM (doxylamine): antihistamine sedative, Rx: insomnia

UNIVASC (moexipril): ACE inhibitor, Rx: HTN

URECHOLINE (bethanechol): cholinergic, Rx: urinary retention

URIMAX (methenamine/salicylate/methylene blue/hyoscyamine): bactericidal, analgesic, antispasmodic, Rx: urinary tract infections

UROXATRAL (alfuzosin): smooth muscle relaxant, Rx: BPH

UROCIT-K (potassium citrate): urinary alkalinizer, Rx: kidney stones
Ursodiol (ACTIGALL): bile acid, Rx: gallstones

V

Valacyclovir (VALTREX): antiviral, Rx: herpes, shingles
VALCYTE (valganciclovir): antiviral, Rx: cytomegalovirus
VALIUM (diazepam): benzodiazepine hypnotic, Rx: anxiety, muscle spasms, seizures, alcohol withdrawal
Valproic acid (DEPAKENE): anticonvulsant, Rx: seizures, migraines, mania
Valrubicin (VALSTAR): antineoplastic, Rx: bladder cancer
Valsartan (DIOVAN): angiotensin II receptor inhibitor, Rx: HTN, CHF, post-MI
VALTREX (valacyclovir): antiviral, Rx: herpes, shingles
VANCOCIN (vancomycin): antibiotic, Rx: bacterial infections
Vancomycin (VANCOCIN): antibiotic, Rx: bacterial infections
VANTIN (cefpodoxime): cephalosporin antibiotic, Rx: bacterial infections
VAPRISOL (conivaptan): increased water excretion, Rx: hyponatremia
VASERETIC (enalapril/HCTZ): ACE inhibitor/diuretic, Rx: HTN
VECTIBIX (panitumamab): antineoplastic, Rx: colorectal cancer
VASOTEC (enalaprilat): ACE inhibitor, Rx: HTN, CHF
VECTIBIX (panitumamab): antineoplastic, Rx: colorectal cancer
Venlafaxine (EFFEXOR): antidepressant, Rx: depression, anxiety, panic disorder
VENOFER (iron sucrose): Rx: iron deficiency anemia in chronic kidney disease and dialysis
VENTOLIN (albuterol): beta$_2$ agonist bronchodilator, Rx: asthma, COPD
Verapamil (CALAN, COVERA-HS, ISOPTIN): calcium channel blocker, Rx: angina, PSVT, HTN
VERELAN, VERELAN PM (verapamil): calcium blocker, Rx: angina, hypertension, PSVT
VERMOX (mebendazole): anthelminthic, Rx: intestinal worms
VESICARE (solifenacin): anticholinergic, Rx: overactive bladder
VFEND (voriconazole): antifungal, Rx: fungal infections
VIAGRA (sildenafil): vasodialator, Rx: male erectile dysfunction
VIBRAMYCIN (doxycycline): tetracycline antibiotic, Rx: bacterial infections

176

VICODIN, VICODIN ES (hydrocodone/APAP): narcotic analgesic compound, Rx: moderate to severe pain

VIDEX (didanosine): antiretroviral, Rx: HIV

VIGAMOX OPTH (moxifloxacin): fluoroquinolone antibiotic, Rx: bacterial conjunctivitis

VIMPAT (lacosamide): anticonvulsant, Rx: partial onset seizure

VIOKASE (pancrelipase): pancreatic enzymes replacement, Rx: chronic pancreatitis, cystic fibrosis

VIRACEPT (nelfinavir): antiretroviral, Rx: HIV

VIRAMUNE (nevirapine): antiretroviral, Rx: HIV

VIREAD (tenofovir): antiretroviral, Rx: HIV, hepatitis B

VISKEN (pindolol): beta blocker, Rx: HTN

VISTARIL (hydroxyzine): antihistamine, Rx: pruritis, sedation, anxiety

VIVELLE (estradiol): transdermal estrogen, Rx: symptoms of menopause

VOLTAREN (diclofenac): NSAID analgesic, Rx: arthritis, pain

VYTORIN (ezetimibe/simvastatin): antihyperlipidemics, Rx: high cholesterol

W

Warfarin (COUMADIN): anticoagulant, Rx: A-Fib, thrombosis

WELCHOL (colesevelam): bile acid sequestrant, Rx: hyperlipidemia

WELLBUTRIN (bupropion): antidepressant, Rx: depression

X

XALATAN OPTH (latanoprost): reduces intraocular pressure, Rx: glaucoma

XANAX, XANAX XR (alprazolam): benzodiazepine, Rx: anxiety disorder, panic attacks

XELODA (capecitabine): antineoplastic, Rx: breast cancer, colorectal cancer

XENICAL (orlistat): lipase inhibitor, Rx: obesity

XIFAXAN (rifaximin): antibiotic, Rx: traveler's diarrhea, hepatic encephalopathy

XOPENEX (levalbuterol): inhaled beta$_2$ bronchodilator, Rx: asthma, COPD

Y

YASMIN 28 (drospirenone/estradiol): oral contraceptive
YAZ (drospirenone/estradiol): oral contraceptive
YODOXIN (iodoquinol): amebicide, Rx: intestinal amebiasis

Z

ZADITOR OPTH (ketotifen): antihistamine, Rx: allergic conjunctivitis
Zaleplon (SONATA): hypnotic, Rx: insomnia
ZANAFLEX (tizanidine): skeletal muscle relaxant
ZARONTIN (ethosuximide): anticonvulsant, Rx: absence seizure
ZAROXOLYN (metolazone): thiazide diuretic, Rx: HTN, fluid retention
ZEBETA (bisoprolol): beta blocker, Rx: HTN
ZEGERID (omeprazole/sodium bicarbonate): proton pump inhibitor compound, Rx: stress ulcer, ulcers, GERD
ZEMPLAR (paricalcitol): vitamin D analog, Rx: hyperparathyroidism in chronic kidney disease
ZERIT (stavudine d4T): antiretroviral, Rx: HIV
ZESTORETIC (lisinopril/HCTZ): ACE inhibitor/diuretic, Rx: HTN
ZESTRIL (lisinopril): ACE inhibitor, Rx: HTN, CHF
ZETIA (ezetimibe): antihyperlipidemic, Rx: hypercholesterolemia
ZIAC (bisoprolol/HCTZ): beta blocker/diuretic, Rx: HTN
ZIAGEN (abacavir): antiretroviral, Rx: HIV
Zidovudine (AZT, RETROVIR): antiretroviral, Rx: HIV
ZINACEF (cefuroxime): cephalosporin antibiotic, Rx: bacterial infections
Zinc oxide: topical protectant, Rx: diaper rash
ZINECARD (dexrazoxane): cardioprotective agent, chelating agent, Rx: cardiomyopathy caused by doxorubicin
ZITHROMAX (azithromycin): macrolide antibiotic, Rx: bacterial infections
ZOCOR (simvastatin): statin, Rx: hypercholesterolemia, CAD
ZOFRAN (ondansetron): 5-HT3 receptor agonist, Rx: nausea and vomiting due to chemotherapy, radiation, and surgery
ZOLADEX (goserelin): gonadotropin-releasing hormone agonist, Rx: endometriosis, prostate cancer, breast cancer
ZOLOFT (sertraline): antidepressant, Rx: depression, OCD, social axiety disorder

Zolpidem (AMBIEM): hypnotic, Rx: insomnia

ZOMETA (zoledronic acid): biphosphonate, Rx: hypercalcemia of malignancy

ZOMIG (zolmitriptan): serotonin receptor agonist, Rx: migraine headache

ZONEGRAN (zonisamide): anticonvulsant, Rx: partial seizures

Zonisamide (ZONEGRAN): anticonvulsant, Rx: partial seizures

ZOSYN (piperacillin/tazobactam): penicillin class antibiotic, Rx: bacterial infections

ZOVIRAX (acyclovir): antiviral, Rx: herpes, shingles, chickenpox

ZYBAN (buproprion): antidepressant, Rx: smoking cessation

ZYFLO (zileuton): bronchospasm inhibitor, Rx: asthma

ZYLOPRIM (allopurinol): xanthine oxidase inhibitor, Rx: gout

ZYMAR OPTH (gatifloxacin): fluoroquinolone, Rx: bacterial conjunctivitis

ZYPREXA, ZYPREXA ZYDIS (olanzapine) antipsychotic, Rx: schizophrenia, bipolar disorder

ZYRTEC (cetirizine): antihistamine, Rx: allergy, hives, asthma

ZYRTEC D (cetirizine/pseudoephedrine): antihistamine/decongestant, Rx: allergic rhinitis

ZYVOX (linezolid): oxazolidinone antibiotic, Rx: bacterial infections

Abbreviations

1°	primary, first degree	**c̄**	with
2°	secondary, second degree	**c/o**	complaining of
3°	tertiary, third degree	**CA**	cancer
≤	less than; less than or equal to	**CAO**	conscious, alert, oriented
≥	greater than; greater than or equal to	**CBG**	capillary blood glucose
≅	approximately equal to	**CHF**	congestive heart failure
α	alpha	**COPD**	chronic obstructive pulmonary disease
ā	before	**CPAP**	continuous positive airway pressure
abd	abdomen	**CVA**	cerebrovascular accident (stroke)
ACE	angiotensin-converting enzyme	**cx**	chest
ADD	attention deficit disorder	**D₅W**	dextrose 5% in water
ADHD	attention deficit/ hyperactivity disorder	**DIC**	disseminated intravascular coagulation
AIDS	acquired immune deficiency syndrome	**dL**	deciliter (1/10 of 1 liter; 100 mL)
AMI	acute myocardial infarction	**DMARD**	disease-modifying antirheumatic drug
APAP	acetaminophen	**DOE**	dyspnea on exertion
APE	acute pulmonary edema	**DSD**	dry sterile dressing
ARC	AIDS related complex	**Dx**	diagnosis
ASA	acetylsalicylic acid (aspirin)	**ECG**	electrocardiogram
β	beta	**ED**	emergency department

180

EPS	extra pyramidal symptoms (dystonias, akathisia, etc.)	IM	intramuscular
ETCO₂	end-tidal carbon dioxide	IO	intraosseous
Fem ♀	female	*Iʊ	*unapproved abbreviation: write out "International Units"
FV	fever	IV	intravenous
Fx	fracture	IVP	IV push
g, gm	gram	IVR	idioventricular rhythm
GCS	Glasgow Coma Scale	K⁺	potassium ion
GI	gastrointestinal	KCl	potassium chloride
gr	grain	kg	kilogram (1,000 grams; 2.2 pounds)
gtt	drop	KVO	keep vein open (30–60 µgtt/minute)
GU	genitourinary	L	liter
H/A	headache	LOC	level of consciousness
HCTZ	hydrochlorothiazide	LP	lumbar puncture
HIV	human immuno-deficiency virus	LUQ	left upper quadrant
H&P	history and physical examintion	min	minute(s)
HR	heart rate	M ♂	male
HTN	hypertension	MAOI	monoamine oxidase inhibitor
Hx	history	mcg	microgram (1/1,000,000 of 1 gram)
ICP	intracranial pressure	MDI	metered dose inhaler
IJR	idiojunctional rhythm	mEq	milliequivalent
IL	intralingual	mg	milligram (1/1,000 of 1 gram)

MI	myocardial infarction	**PR**	per rectum; rectally
mL	milliliter (1/1,000 of 1 liter; 1 mL)	**PSVT**	paroxysmal supra-ventricular tachycardia
~~**ms**~~	write out morphine	**PVC**	premature ventricular contraction
~~**MSO₄**~~	write out morphine sulfate	**q̄**	every
NaHCO₃	sodium bicarbonate	**RL**	Ringer's lactate
N&V, N/V	nausea and vomiting	**RR**	respiratory rate
NAD	no acute distress, no apparent distress	**Rx**	prescribed for, used for
NG	nasogastric	**s̄**	without
NR	Normosol–R	**s/s**	signs and symptoms
NS	normal saline (0.9% NaCl)	**SaO₂**	arterial oxygen saturation
NSAID	non-steroidal anti-inflammatory drug	**ScvO2**	central venous oxygen saturation
NTG	nitroglycerin	**SL**	sublingual
OLMC	On-Line Medical Control	**SOB**	shortness of breath, dyspnea
p̄	after	**SQ**	subcutaneous
PCP	pneumocystis carinii	**SW**	sterile water
PETCO₂	partial pressure of end-tidal carbon dioxide	**Sz**	seizure
PO	by mouth, orally	**TB**	tuberculosis
POC	position of comfort	**TCA**	tricyclic antidepressant
prn	as needed	**TKO**	to keep open (30–60 μgtt/minute)

Torr	millimeters mercury (mm Hg)	WPW	Wolff-Parkinson-White (syndrome)
*U̶	*write out "unit"	x	times
URI	upper respiratory infection	↓	decreased
UTI	urinary tract infection	↑	increased
UV	umbilical vein, ultraviolet	μ	micro (1/1,000,000)
VF	ventricular fibrillation	Δ	change (delta)
VNS	vagus nerve stimulator	⊘	no, none, null
VT	ventricular tachycardia		

Notes

Phone Numbers

911 Communications Center
American Red Cross
Chemtrec Emergency # 1-800-424-9300
Chemtrec Non-emergency # 1-800-262-8200
Children's Services
CISD Team
Crisis Center
Domestic Violence Shelter
HazMat Team
Homeless Shelter
Medical Examiner/Coroner
Medical Resource Hospital
National Response Center # 1-800-424-8802
Poison Control Center
Public Health Department
Sexual Abuse/Rape Victim Hotline
State/County EMS Office
Translation Services
Trauma Center
Other

Notes